Francis G. Caro, PhD
Editor

Family and Aging Policy

Family and Aging Policy has been co-published simultaneously as *Journal of Aging & Social Policy*, Volume 18, Numbers 3/4 2006.

Pre-publication
REVIEWS,
COMMENTARIES,
EVALUATIONS . . .

"**F**inally, there is a book that addresses, in one volume, the critical issues in aging policy as it relates to family and family caregiving. The authors SKILLFULLY TACKLE A WIDE RANGE OF ISSUES including values, laws, and housing and family caregiver intervention programs. Moving from a focus on international perspectives to a focus on US Policy and Local variations in local implementation and practice, the book EXAMINES BOTH INTENTIONAL AND UNINTENTIONAL LINKS BETWEEN PUBLIC POLICIES AND FAMILY WELL-BEING. In combination, the chapters clearly articulate the ambivalence toward the family that is present in public policy and public program affecting elders. At the same time, the book makes clear the link between quality elder care and family well-being. This volume is SURE TO BECOME A CORE STAPLE FOR COURSES ON FAMILY AND LONG TERM CARE AND ON AGING POLICY."

Rhonda J.V. Montgomery, PhD,
Helen Bader Endowed Chair
in Applied Gerontology
Department of Sociology &
Helen Bader School of Social Welfare
University of Wisconsin-Milwaukee

More pre-publication
REVIEWS, COMMENTARIES, EVALUATIONS . . .

"This eclectic monograph includes thirteen VERY TIMELY, EMPIRICAL articles, each positioned at a slightly different angle to the nexus of family policy and aging policy. . . . Policy critiques from Sweden, Denmark, Singapore and Canada highlight a range of policies–and policy lacunae–between absolutist positions favoring family *or* government responsibility. Each author addresses a unique aspect of a middle road; neither "the family" nor "the government" can, or should, "do it all." Reality poses both more opportunities and more challenges than can be met with simplistic solutions. I HEARTILY RECOMMEND THIS BOOK as a supplemental text for graduate courses in Social Work, Family Studies, Social Policy, and especially, Aging Policy. . . . This affordable volume OFFERS CRITICAL ANALYSES OF RICH TOPICS OF CURRENT INTEREST to practitioners as well as policymakers of all ideological stripes."

Sharon Keigher, PhD, Professor
Helen Bader School of Social Welfare
University of Wisconsin-Milwaukee

"AN IMPORTANT CONTRIBUTION to the field of family caregiving. It gathers in one place a series of articles highlighting various aspects of public policy that both directly and indirectly affect the financial, emotional and physical capacity of families to care for their elders. . . . Provides readers with A WEALTH OF INFORMATION from international as well as domestic experiences, adding new insights into the strengths of and gaps in the American system. In particular, this series of articles underscores the lack of a coherent family policy in the United States and its failure, with some exceptions (e.g., the Family and Medical Leave Act), to recognize elder care as a crucial part of public policy across the family life span. One of the strengths of this volume is that it addresses several policy areas that have not to date received adequate attention. These include the implications of zoning regulations for co-residential family caregiving, the impact of welfare reform on grandparents as caregivers, and the effects of state policy decisions on the financial well-being of later-life families. The breadth and scope of this new book will provide IMPORTANT NEW INSIGHTS into and a better understanding of the connections between public policy and the ability of our major long-term care provider–the family–to care for an aging society."

Robyn I. Stone, Dr. PH
Executive Director of the Institute
for the Future of Aging Services
American Association of Homes
and Services for the Aging

The Haworth Press, Inc.

New York • London • Victoria (AU)
www.HaworthPress.com

Family and Aging Policy

Family and Aging Policy has been co-published simultaneously as *Journal of Aging & Social Policy*, Volume 18, Numbers 3/4 2006.

Family and Aging Policy, edited by Francis G. Caro, PhD (Vol. 18, No. 3/4, 2006). *"Finally, there is a book that addresses, in one volume, the critical issues in aging policy as it relates to family and family caregiving. The authors SKILLFULLY TACKLE A WIDE RANGE OF ISSUES. . . . SURE TO BECOME A CORE STAPLE FOR COURSES ON FAMILY AND LONG TERM CARE AND ON AGING POLICY." (Rhonda J. V. Montgomery, PhD, Helen Bader Endowed Chair in Applied Gerontology, Department of Sociology & Helen Bader School of Social Welfare, University of Wisconsin-Milwaukee)*

An Aging India: Perspectives, Prospects, and Policies, edited by Phoebe S. Liebig, PhD, and S. Irudaya Rajan, PhD (Vol. 15, No. 2/3, 2003). *"The most definitive collection on this subject . . . . A major achievement. . . . Remarkable for its breadth, its intellectual depth, and most of all for its consistent readability. . . . A valuable addition for all scholars and planners working in this field." (Indrani Chakravarty, PhD, Director, Calcutta Metropolitan Institute of Gerontology)*

Devolution and Aging Policy, edited by Francis G. Caro, PhD, and Robert Morris, DSW (Vol. 14, No. 3/4, 2002). *Examines devolution–the decentralizing of service provision–and roles that state/local government and private organizations now play in addressing the needs of elders.*

Long-Term Care in the 21st Century: Perspectives from Around the Asia-Pacific Rim, edited by Iris Chi, DSW, Kalyani K. Mehta, PhD, and Anna L. Howe, PhD (Vol. 13, No. 2/3, 2001). *Discusses policies and programs for long-term care in the United States, Canada, Japan, Australia, Singapore, Hong Kong, and Taiwan.*

Advancing Aging Policy as the 21st Century Begins, edited by Francis G. Caro, PhD, Robert Morris, DSW, and Jill Norton (Vol. 11, No. 2/3, 2000). *"An ideal textbook for any graduate-level course on the aging population. Stands out among existing books on social problems and policies of the aging society. Succinct and to the point. A must-read for students, researchers, policy advocates, and policymakers." (Namkee G. Choi, PhD, Professor, Portland State University, Oregon)*

Public Policy and the Old Age Revolution in Japan, edited by Scott A. Bass, PhD, Robert Morris, DSW, and Masato Oka, MSc (Vol. 8, No. 2/3, 1996). *"Anyone seriously interested in the 21st Century and exploring means of adaptation to the revolution in longevity should read this book." (Robert N. Butler, MD, Director, International Longevity Center, The Mount Sinai Medical Center, New York)*

From Nursing Homes to Home Care, edited by Marie E. Cowart, DrPH, and Jill Quadagno, PhD (Vol. 7, No. 3/4, 1996). *"A compendium of research and policy information related to long-term care services, aging, and disability. Contributors address topics encompassing the risk of disability, access to and need for long-term care, and planning for a future long-term care policy." (Family Caregiver Alliance)*

International Perspectives on State and Family Support for the Elderly, edited by Scott A. Bass, PhD, and Robert Morris, DSW (Vol. 5, No. 1/2, 1993). *"The cross-cultural perspectives of the volume and the questions asked about what services are really needed and by whom they should be provided will be useful to the authors' intended audience in gerontological policymaking." (Academic Library Book Review)*

Family and Aging Policy

Francis G. Caro, PhD
Editor

Family and Aging Policy has been co-published simultaneously as
Journal of Aging & Social Policy, Volume 18, Numbers 3/4 2006.

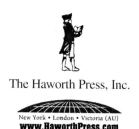

The Haworth Press, Inc.

New York • London • Victoria (AU)
www.HaworthPress.com

Family and Aging Policy has been co-published simultaneously as *Journal of Aging & Social Policy*™, Volume 18, Numbers 3/4 2006.

Library of Congress Cataloging-in-Publication Data

Family and aging policy / Francis G. Caro, editor.
    p. cm.
    "Family and Aging Policy has been co-published simultaneously as Journal of Aging & Social Policy, Volume 18, Numbers 3/4 2006."
    Includes bibliographical references and index.
    ISBN-13: 978-0-7890-3373-4 (hard cover : alk. paper)
    ISBN-10: 0-7890-3373-9 (hard cover : alk. paper)
    ISBN-13: 978-0-7890-3374-1 (soft cover : alk. paper)
    ISBN-10: 0-7890-3374-7 (soft cover : alk. paper)
    1. Older people–Government policy–United States. 2. Aging parents–Care–United States. 3. Caregivers–Services for United States. 4. Older people–Government policy–Case studies. I. Caro, Francis G., 1936- II. Journal of aging & social policy.
  HV1461.F33 2006
  362.6–dc22
                              2006029976

Indexing, Abstracting & Website/Internet Coverage

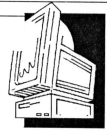

This section provides you with a list of major indexing & abstracting services and other tools for bibliographic access. That is to say, each service began covering this periodical during the year noted in the right column. Most Websites which are listed below have indicated that they will either post, disseminate, compile, archive, cite or alert their own Website users with research-based content from this work. (This list is as current as the copyright date of this publication.)

(continued)

(continued)

(continued)

*Exact start date to come.

*Special Bibliographic Notes related to special journal issues
(separates) and indexing/abstracting:*

- indexing/abstracting services in this list will also cover material in any "separate" that is co-published simultaneously with Haworth's special thematic journal issue or DocuSerial. Indexing/abstracting usually covers material at the article/chapter level.
- monographic co-editions are intended for either non-subscribers or libraries which intend to purchase a second copy for their circulating collections.
- monographic co-editions are reported to all jobbers/wholesalers/approval plans. The source journal is listed as the "series" to assist the prevention of duplicate purchasing in the same manner utilized for books-in-series.
- to facilitate user/access services all indexing/abstracting services are encouraged to utilize the co-indexing entry note indicated at the bottom of the first page of each article/chapter/contribution.
- this is intended to assist a library user of any reference tool (whether print, electronic, online, or CD-ROM) to locate the monographic version if the library has purchased this version but not a subscription to the source journal.
- individual articles/chapters in any Haworth publication are also available through the Haworth Document Delivery Service (HDDS).

Family and Aging Policy

CONTENTS

THE UNITED STATES

ABOUT THE EDITOR

Francis G. Caro, PhD, is Professor of Gerontology at the University of Massachusetts Boston. He received a PhD in Sociology from the University of Minnesota. Dr. Caro's major current research interests are organization of home and community-based long-term care for elders, planning of residential adjustments associated with the aging process, and productive aging. He is the editor of the *Journal of Aging & Social Policy* and co-editor of a number of books including *Devolution and Aging* (2002), *Advancing Aging Policy as the 21st Century Begins* (2000), and *Achieving a Productive Aging Society* (1993). In addition, he is a co-author of *Personal Assistance: The Future of Home Care, Quality Impact of Home Care for the Elderly* (1988), and *Family Care of the Elderly* (1981). He edited *Readings in Evaluation Research* (1977). Dr. Caro teaches policy courses in the graduate programs in Gerontology at the University of Massachusetts Boston.

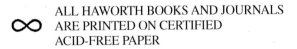

INTRODUCTION

Family and Aging Policy

Francis G. Caro, PhD

Gerontology Institute, University of Massachusetts Boston

Historically, in "advanced" societies the emergence of public interventions to address special needs of elders can be traced to the limitations of families. In earlier eras in these societies, families were the primary source of assistance for dependent elders. In those times, the vast majority of those who survived to old age lived within multigenerational households. In part, public interventions to assist dependent elders in advanced societies are a reflection of the fact that both extended and nuclear families have weakened. Significant numbers of elders do not have relatives to call upon when they need assistance. Public interventions also have their origins in some substantial needs of elders that greatly exceed the capacity of families to provide help. (Other major factors also contributed to the emergence of significant public sector intervention including economic development, which has provided the financial underpinnings.)

[Haworth co-indexing entry note]: "Family and Aging Policy." Caro, Francis G. Co-published simultaneously in *Journal of Aging & Social Policy* (The Haworth Press, Inc.) Vol. 18, No. 3/4, 2006, pp. 1-5; and: *Family and Aging Policy* (ed: Francis G. Caro) The Haworth Press, Inc., 2006, pp. 1-5. Single or multiple copies of this article are available for a fee from The Haworth Document Delivery Service [1-800-HAWORTH, 9:00 a.m. - 5:00 p.m. (EST). E-mail address: docdelivery@haworthpress.com].

Available online at http://jasp.haworthpress.com
doi:10.1300/J031v18n03_01

The family ties of elders in advanced societies are varied and highly complex. Elders who have no significant family involvement are the exception. For the majority of older people, many aspects of the aging experience tend to unfold in a family context. Examples of the family and aging connection are abundant. The timing of retirement is often the reflection of the agenda of married couples. For elders who are married, financial security is a reflection of joint income and assets. For married elders who co-reside with their spouses, housing choices are choices of couples (and sometimes other family members). For elders who co-reside with adult children, housing is a multigenerational family matter. For elders who need long-term care, unpaid relatives tend to be the first source of care and the most important source of long-term care. Family members are often involved with elders in negotiating the health care system. These examples illustrate the fact that, in the key areas of income security, housing, long-term care, and health care, the welfare of individual elders is often a reflection of their family circumstances.

The manner in which public programs affecting elders take families into account is varied. Some public programs are directly focused on families. In the United States, the Social Security Act, for example, was designed to protect both individual workers and their families. In addition to providing pensions for disabled and retired workers, the Social Security program provides pension benefits for survivors of deceased workers and spouses of retired workers. The Family Medical Leave Act is another example of a public intervention with an explicit family focus. The Act makes it possible for employees to take unpaid leave under certain circumstance in order to provide assistance to family members. Another example is the family caregiver provisions of the Older Americans Act that are designed to provide assistance to informal providers of long-term care.

Other public programs serving elders are focused on individuals but have important implications for families. Medicaid, for example, is fundamentally a source of health care financing for individuals. At the same time, Medicaid includes some explicit provisions concerning families. For elders who are seeking Medicaid-financed nursing home care, assets jointly owned by married couples pose a complication in determination of financial eligibility. Medicaid administrative policy addresses issues concerned with the complications associated with taking into account assets jointly owned by married couples in determining individual eligibility.

Historically, Medicaid has also addressed questions about the responsibility of adult children to pay for long-term care for their aging parents. The filial responsibility issue has important financial implications for relatives. Public payment for nursing home care relieves family members of the obligation to pay for care.

Medicaid policy has also taken a position on the hiring of immediate family members as providers of financed care. On a long-standing basis, Medicaid programs have prohibited the hiring of immediate family members as personal assistance providers financed through Medicaid. Some contemporary consumer-directed care programs have challenged this long-standing policy.

The reasons for examining the implications of aging policy for families are multiple. One reason is to evaluate the direct effects of policies designed to affect families. When policies are designed to support families engaged in eldercare, for example, questions can be asked about their vertical and horizontal efficiency, that is, the extent to which they reach those in need of support and the extent of need among those who do receive assistance. Also of interest is the effectiveness of interventions in assisting those who use them. The indirect effects of family policies for individual elders also deserve attention. Of particular interest are instances in which the welfare of elders and families are in conflict.

Another reason to pursue this topic is to examine indirect implications for families of policies designed to affect individual elders. These effects may be unanticipated. Policies that limit the scope of public financing of services for elders, for example, often have financial implications for families when families become the payers of last resort because of inadequacy of public financing.

In the United States, possibilities for widespread indirect effects of policy on families are abundant because of the many aspects of policy that can affect elders, the narrow scope of many policies, and the absence of an explicit public policy agenda either for elders or their families. Individual elders and their families are expected to solve their own problems except in the exceptional situations in which the public sector has chosen to intervene. The situation is further complicated by the fact that the public sector can intervene at the federal, state, or local level.

Questions about the interplay between public interventions and families on aging issues arise in every country with some level of public attention to the needs of elders. Internationally, variation in the scope of public-sector intervention on needs of elders is enormous. In many developing countries, public intervention is nominal; extended families remain the mainstay in support of dependent elders. In more developed countries, the public interventions are often at least as well developed as they are in the United States. At the same time, the involvement of families in elder support issues is extensive in all of these countries. Consequently, the potential for complex interaction between families and public interventions is great.

The papers in this volume are responses to a widely circulated call for papers. The intent was to include papers on many aspects of aging and policy that drew upon experiences in the United States and elsewhere. We succeeded in attracting a strong international response with four articles on experiences in countries other than the United States. Most of the papers are concerned with the role of family in providing long-term care. The heavy emphasis on this topic is not surprising in light of the major role that families play in providing care to elders living in the community and the fact that public programs tend to operate as supplements to informal care.

All but one of the papers are concerned with aspects of caregiving. Of the 12 articles concerned with caregiving, 11 are focused on elder care. The other paper deals with grandparents who care for their grandchildren. The volume begins with the articles on elder care. We have placed the papers on Sweden, Denmark, Singapore, and Canada first because they demonstrate effectively the universality of the tension between family and public responsibility for elder care. In each of these countries, families willingly play the major role in long-term care. The demands of caregiving often exceed the capacity of family members to provide all of the care that is needed. In every case, families look to the public sector for assistance. The manner in which the public sector complements family caregiving varies from one country to another. Lennarth Johannsson and Gerdt Sundström provide a historical perspective on shifts in the manner in which filial obligations have changed over time in Sweden. They argue that intergenerational solidarity in Sweden remains strong in spite of the country's extensive welfare programs. Similarly, Mary Stuart and Eigil Boll Hansen report that, in Denmark, even with the introduction of extensive publicly-funded home care programs for elders, involvement of family caregivers remains extensive. Examining family-oriented social policies of the Singapore government, Kalyani K. Mehta argues that the government should do more to help family caregivers look after elder relatives. Reporting on a study conducted in Quebec, Canada, Nancy Guberman and colleagues examine shared responsibilities of families and formal services for frail elders. They find high expectations for family caregiving at the same time that they find strong support for publicly-funded programs to support caregivers.

The papers about caregiving in the United States begin with an account by Lynn Friss Feinberg and Sandra L. Newman of the early experiences of the Administration on Aging's National Family Caregiver Support program. We follow with two papers concerned with employment and elder care. Donna L. Wagner provides a broad examination of employment and elder care. Steven Wisensale then argues for paid leave as a means of strengthening the Family Medical Leave Act. Carol J. Whitlatch and Lynn Friss Feinberg examine the experiences of California Caregiver Resource Centers that permit families to hire relatives and friends as in-home respite providers. Looking at the fact that eldercare responsibilities often continue for a number of years and change over time, Joseph E. Gaugler and Pamela Teaster examine the implications for policy and community-based care programs. Phoebe S. Liebig, Teresa Koenig, and Jon Pynoos call attention to the role of accessory dwelling units in facilitating family caregiving. They demonstrate the importance of local zoning ordinances in enabling this form of intergenerational co-residence. Carrie A. Levin and Rosalie A. Kane show that in assisted living, residents and family members have distinct perspectives on the features offered by facilities.

In her article about grandparents raising grandchildren, Casey E. Copen shows how welfare reform has affected intergenerational households headed by grandparents.

In the final article, Gretchen J. Hill examines the manner in which changes in state rules during the 1990s affected such areas as inheritance, estate taxes, homestead exemptions, Medicaid eligibility, and estate recovery. Hill's article is important in showing that public policy concerning families goes far beyond caregiving issues.

INTERNATIONAL VIEW

Policies and Practices
in Support of Family Caregivers–
Filial Obligations Redefined in Sweden

Lennarth Johansson, PhD

Socialstyrelsen, Stockholm, Sweden

Gerdt Sundström, PhD

School of Health Sciences, Jönköping, Sweden

SUMMARY. This article provides an overview of how the expression of filial obligations has shifted over time in Sweden. Historically, and currently in many countries, the family, next of kin, and the social network are the only or major sources of help, as it was in Sweden till half a century ago. The article also explores how various aspects of solidarity–public and private–have developed and are changing in Sweden, known for its extensive welfare programs, with "from cradle to grave" security. It

[Haworth co-indexing entry note]: "Policies and Practices in Support of Family Caregivers–Filial Obligations Redefined in Sweden."Johansson, Lennarth, and Gerdt Sundström. Co-published simultaneously in *Journal of Aging & Social Policy* (The Haworth Press, Inc.) Vol. 18, No. 3/4, 2006, pp. 7-26; and: *Family and Aging Policy* (ed: Francis G. Caro) The Haworth Press, Inc., 2006, pp. 7-26. Single or multiple copies of this article are available for a fee from The Haworth Document Delivery Service [1-800-HAWORTH, 9:00 a.m. - 5:00 p.m. (EST). E-mail address: docdelivery@haworthpress.com].

Available online at http://jasp.haworthpress.com
doi:10.1300/J031v18n03_02   7

concludes that intergenerational solidarity has not vanished in Sweden; just the manifestations have changed. doi:10.1300/J031v18n03_02

[Article copies available for a fee from The Haworth Document Delivery Service: 1-800-HAWORTH. E-mail address: <docdelivery@haworthpress.com> Website: <http://www.HaworthPress.com> © 2006 by The Haworth Press, Inc. All rights reserved.]

KEYWORDS. Old age care, family, public services, Home Help

INTRODUCTION

The expression of filial obligations has shifted over time and varies internationally. Historically, and currently in many countries, the family, next of kin, and the social network at large have been and are the only or major sources of help, as it was in Sweden till half a century ago. One may say that dependent elderly persons rely on an implicit intergenerational contract, guaranteeing necessary support on a normative basis. In this sense, changes in care provided within the family and social network indicate a normative change in patterns of relations and exchanges between individuals, what we often term "solidarity."

Patterns of care for the elderly have received increasing attention over the last three decades, in Sweden and elsewhere. The reasons are well-known: More elders and more elders who live alone and need help. The explanations given for these changes vary, from purely demographic trends–the many elders who "overburden" shrinking families and the state–to the "disappearance" of the housewife, shifts in norms and values, social atomization, and waning filial piety. Others argue that intergenerational solidarity has not vanished, but that the manifestations have changed. Help to parents and other kin was never unconditional, not even when stipulated in law.

All the disintegrative forces are presumed to have culminated in Nordic welfare states, but they are well under way in many other societies. In Europe, several countries have legally binding filial obligations (Millar & Warman, 1996). The Nordic countries never had these obligations (Denmark) or recently abolished them. Other countries (e.g., Germany and France) seem to apply them only when institutional care is the option. In many welfare states, public spending may have reached a ceiling, as tax increases are politically impossible, and the issue then is how best to use available resources. Countries with fewer extensive public services tend to focus more on economic support and pensions, though the picture is complex and does not always concur with the wishes of carers. For example, a recent (2004) nationwide Spanish survey of carers found that they above all want services, and more now than 10 years earlier. Financial support is less asked for, but still important because many carers suffer financially from their commitment (IMSERSO, 2004). The Nordic countries have invested more in services and residential care, though financial support has been used as well, but frequently as a secondary and marginal strategy.

With some guidance by a theory on intergenerational solidarity (Bengtson & Roberts, 1991), this article explores how various aspects of solidarity–public and private–have developed and are changing in Sweden, known for its extensive welfare programs, with "from cradle to grave" security. The sustainability and consequences of these policies might be of interest for American policymakers.

FILIAL AND PUBLIC OBLIGATIONS–A SYMBIOTIC STORY

Public responsibility for the frail, poor, and elderly has a very long tradition in the Nordic countries. There, the poor tithe was, by special permission, gathered and spent locally after collective decisions in the parishes in medieval times, rather then being forwarded to the ecclesiastical hierarchy as on the continent. The significance of this heritage is often overlooked, perhaps because these structures took form so early. Parish meetings on poor-relief and other communal affairs later developed into municipal councils (1862). These, together with village meetings, road maintenance associations, a court system with locally elected laymen, various self-help organizations, non-conformist religious groups, tea-totallers, labor unions and political organizations, library associations, and other more or less formalized citizen fora became so much part of Swedish life that they are now taken for granted. Yet, it remains that many modern welfare programs started out early, on a voluntary basis. The legal responsibility of the parish-municipality for their paupers, formalized in 1788, was of great importance because it trained (the more affluent) locals to take part in communal problem-solving and, early on, established habits of compromise and trust (in short, "social capital"). It also fostered the perception that care for the poor and elderly (often the same persons) was a concern both communally and locally. The Nordic welfare state has an old foundation and in a way, it's just the scope of action that is much larger today.

Inheritance rules and the corresponding expectation that heirs would provide care were stipulated in medieval laws in Sweden but applied only to the relatively well-to-do. In the early 1700s, a system (*undantag*) emerged where farmers (or other landowners) could transfer their property at a reduced price to offspring (or anyone else) and in return have a guarantee of food, shelter, and care, typically including a decent burial. The property served as security in contracts, which often specified the tribute in great detail. An 18th century law that required people without a livelihood to find an employer (vagrants were often arrested and sent to forced labor) made exceptions for women caring for frail parents. Still, in 1954, 6% of the Swedish elderly lived with *undantag-contract*–vanished today, but still surviving in Finland and Norway.

One should not romanticize the local provision of relief to the poor. Parishioners were generally poor, and human shortcomings sometimes interfered with provisions that, at best, were patriarchal and in the spirit of almsgiving. In spite of repeated central instructions over the centuries regarding what should be done, local differences in provision persisted and were still large in 1829, as disclosed in a government survey that year (Skoglund, 1992). Tensions between a powerful state and a semi-autonomous periphery have long roots in the Nordic countries.

After stipulating municipal obligations for the poor, filial duties were established. The poor-relief board in the parish, before giving any help, had to consider "the responsibility to see to the needs of the poor person that could be tied to kin or other persons" (Poor Relief Regulation, SFS 23, 1847 para. 4), though conditioned by their ability to provide. It is easy to find cases in the poor relief records where family members evaded the task with impunity or where they did provide, but received money from the poor relief board to alleviate their burden. There were obligations both on the public side and on kin's side.

In 1855 a government resolution restricted obligations to parent-child, a clause that remained in poor laws till 1956. Filial obligations were abolished in Swedish civil law in 1979 with explicit reference to pensions and old-age care now being so adequate that these regulations were obsolete. The lawmakers at the same time found it appropriate to point out that they in no way wanted to abolish the "moral obligation by offspring to help and support their parents in other ways."

By the early 1800s, Swedish poor relief clients could appeal local decisions in their cases to the county governor's office. The legal right to appeal decisions in old-age care free-of-charge up through the ladder of administrative courts was established in the Social Service Act of 1982. Yet, complaints on old-age care are rare, and probably less common than they should be. The County Administrative Board acts on complaints, inspects, and strives to supervise residential care and home-based care for the elderly.

CHANGING OLD-AGE CARE IN SWEDEN

In modern times, Sweden and the other Nordic countries gradually replaced the intergenerational contract with a societal contract. Indeed, one of the explicit cornerstones in the post-war Swedish welfare system was to substitute public services for former family responsibilities. In pace with the economic growth, the state should gradually extend services and care for children, the disabled, and the elderly. In that vein, from the 1960s and up to the second half of the1980s, public old-age care expanded substantially in the Nordic countries.

Before 1950, public old-age care in Sweden equaled poor relief and often meant institutional care. About 20% of those aged 80 years and older were institutionalized in 1950. Major scandals in old-age homes and public pressure by media and demands from the fledgling pensioners' movements forced the government instead to promote public Home Help (help with chores but also personal care), that expanded dramatically in the next two decades. Yet, institutionalization also grew rapidly. In 1975, 30% of those 80 and older in Sweden were institutionalized, and 39% used public Home Help, that is, 7 out of 10 were covered (Sundström, Johansson, & Hassing, 2002). By that time, fees were low or waived altogether, and in all fairness it may be said that there was a degree of over-consumption of services.

In 2003, 19% of those 80 years and older were institutionalized and the same proportion used public Home Help; together these services covered 4 out of 10 of those 80 years and older. These are national averages: local variations in services for the elderly were and are big, in Sweden. Help to elders living in the community has suffered most during the 1990s. Institutional care is, by nature, more difficult to cut back or to run at half speed, but beginning around the year 2000, substantial cutbacks have also been made in institutional coverage. In general, cutbacks were accompanied by stricter and more professional needs-assessments, which tend to follow the letter of the law: services are provided "when a need cannot be seen to by other means."

In the 1970s-1980s, according to one study, about half of the elderly died without having ever used any public service. In recent studies, rates are much lower: Today, 90-95% of elders eventually seem to use public old-age care. Prevalence rates (in cross-sectional statistics) may decrease and incidence rates may rise simultaneously. One might interpret the above findings as improved targeting, but it comes at a cost: Elders now use help later and for a shorter period of time. Evidence of this is not collected routinely; therefore, cross-sectional data are used in Table 1 to describe changing support patterns. Public services may have decreased for a number of reasons. Municipalities are hard pressed financially, and there are budget restrictions, since Sweden already has the world's highest tax rates. Two thirds of all personal tax is paid to and spent by the municipalities, which are nearly self-financed and constitutionally independent. Government attempts to prescribe what municipalities should do–without providing sufficient means–are countered by municipal rationing and/or watering down of the quality of the services.

Some elderly tend to refrain from or postpone the use of these services when co-payments are raised, but fees also induce users to demand quality, which they increasingly do. Others, particularly those more well off, find it to their advantage instead to buy private services or to remunerate family for help given. Further, raised standards of living of successive cohorts of the elderly may also decrease dependence

TABLE 1. Family Care, Public Home Help, and Institutional Care for Elders, Sweden, 1954, 1975, 1994, and 2000

		Year			
		1954	1975	1994	2000
	Age	67+	65+	75+	75+
Received support from family*[1]		77%	39%	34%	37%
	65+[1]	1%	17%	9%	8%
Home help	75+[2]	..	..	18%	15%
	80+[1]	..	39%	22%	20%
Institutional care	80+	20%	30%	23%	21%

[1] percentage of total population.
[2] percentage of community-residing elders.
* All kinds of relatives, including small numbers of friends and neighbors, helping with household chores (1954). In 1975, 1994, and 2000, also personal care (see footnote of Table 2), but very few received help with this only.
Source: Johansson, Sundström, & Hassing, 2003.

on public support. As implied, rationing of services can be compatible with improved targeting in the longer run. This may be seen as a system response in a situation where it is impossible to expand service coverage.

Old-age care in the Nordic countries is in practice a municipal monopoly, with one point entry where all needs assessments and eligibility issues are handled by the same case manager. A good deal of the success of the system and its viability in the present situation of cutbacks is due to the simplicity of the system and its local anchorage, administratively and in day-to-day work.

To sum up, the Swedish welfare state has retreated and a similar process seems to be under way in the other Nordic countries. For mainly economic reasons, the expansion was halted in Sweden in the 1990s; after that, coverage ratios of various services have dropped substantially. This, then, points in the direction of a more selective mode of welfare provision. Previous fears that the state would eventually crowd out all family care were unfounded. In 1950, about 5% of the Swedish GDP was spent on the elderly (pensions, housing allowances, old-age homes, etc.); since the 1990s, the proportion is about 12%, and government budget forecasts show that it will not increase in the near future. When public services cannot keep up with demands for care, there remains the family or other private initiatives—or that (some) needy persons live in misery.

FAMILY CARE IN SWEDEN

In the 1990s, the family and family care was "re-discovered" in elder care in Sweden and even found its way into legislation. There are several explanations of this. First, one of the major experiences in promoting home-based community care was that home care is often dependent on extensive family caregiving. Second, along with the economic recession, there has been a growing interest in the informal care sector and its potential to substitute for costly formal services. Third, in recent years there is also increasing research evidence pointing to the crucial role of families, their care commitments, and their ensuing need for support. Fourthly, and most recently, carers and their organizations are now more openly lobbying for recognition and support. The resulting effect is a growing awareness that support for carers is a necessary precondition to mobilize carers in the future, which in turn is of crucial importance for the whole system of elderly welfare in an era of shrinking public services. In a more critical vein, one might say that public recognition of family caregiving was very timely, as it coincided with the welfare program cutbacks.

As shown in Table 1, family care decreased steeply from the early 1950s, but then leveled off and seems to have increased somewhat in the 1990s (the 1994 and 2000 studies exactly comparable). Much help in the 1950s and 1960s concerned tasks like wood-chopping and water-carrying, no longer needed since 99% of the Swedish elderly now have modern housing, compared to about 20% in 1954 and 80% in 1975. Generally speaking, modern housing and adequate pensions facilitate independent living. Surveys also indicate that this increasingly is the preference.

Also, by other measures family care did increase in the 1990s: families are estimated to have provided 60% of all community care in 1994, but 70% in 2000, for elders 75 + (Sundström, Johansson, & Hassing, 2002). Since there are nearly three times more old people today than in 1950, this implies an absolute increase in family care. Likewise, a thorough Norwegian study found no evidence that the state had replaced family care (Lingsom, 1997). Spouses and adult children provide most of this family support, and there are more of both. More old people have children and more are married and also stay married longer, with a vast increase in Golden Weddings and other long-lived marriages, in spite of a simultaneous rise in elderly divorces.

Counter intuitively, men care for wives about as much as women care for husbands; many men need no help before they die, or only little help for a short time (Sundström et al., 2003). More elders are married: In the age-group 80+, 20% were married in 1950, as against 32% in year 2002. Of all the elderly 65+, 54% are married and another 4% co-habit with a partner. Further, maybe 7% of the elderly have partners with whom they do not live; that is, they are "living apart together" (Tornstam, 2005). The care provided by adult children is described in some detail in Table 2. Help from family, in particular children, increased in the 1990s.

The state can support caring families *directly*, but also *indirectly* through services: Offspring are relieved when aging parents use Home Help. Direct support to family carers is unusual in Sweden, with indirect support through the public Home Help decreasing. Yet, this service is the dominant source of help for Swedish elders with neither spouse nor children (it provides both household help and personal care, though it strives to restrict itself to the latter). Home Help clients pay a fee, according to income and number of hours used, up to a ceiling. The average client uses 32 hours/month, with large variations and no upper limit.

TABLE 2. Care for Elderly People 75+ Who Live Alone, Help from Children*
and from Public Home Help. Sweden 1994 and 2000

Year	All 1994	All 2000	Has offspring, all elders 1994	Has offspring, all elders 2000	Offspring within 15 km 1994	Offspring within 15 km 2000	Childless 1994	Childless 2000
Help from Children	12%	22%	16%	28%	16%	36%	–	–
Home Help	25%	20%	24%	18%	23%	19%	27%	29%
N (weighted)	716	843	547	670	371	414	170	173

Note: Home Help is a needs-assessed public service that in Sweden provides help with *household tasks* (primarily shopping, cooking, cleaning, and laundry) and/or with *personal care* (getting into/out-of bed, bathing, toileting, eating, un/dressing, outdoor walks, etc.).
*Both for Home Help and children, help refers to aid with one or more of these aspects.
Sources: Johansson, Sundström, & Hassing, 2003.

Four percent of all Home Help recipients use more than 120 hours/
month.

Currently, in Sweden, only *married* persons have legal obligations to
support their partners, though this officially does not include "heavy"
personal care. As indicated, the Social Service Act states that a municipality has an obligation to provide help if a need cannot be seen to otherwise. This has recently been interpreted, with dubious legality, to the
effect that elders who have offspring or other family living nearby or
who are well-to-do are denied public help. In a way, this reminds us of
the situation half a century ago when public services equaled poor relief. As mentioned, filial obligations then applied, as they still do in
many European countries. Some potential users are now instead helped
by family, or they buy private services. In the 1970s and 1980s, there
were no class differences in the use of public home help, but such
differences seem to have reemerged.

Patterns of living and care are closely related. In contemporary Sweden the elderly and their adult children rarely live together; about 2% do
so. This is also gradually decreasing in most other European countries,
though Italy seems to be an exception. The Swedish elderly live alone
(40% of those 65 years and older) or–importantly–with just their spouse/
partner. Solitary living has culminated at least in the Nordic countries,
in the Netherlands, and in Britain. It is less common, but increasing, in
Southern Europe. Yet, family should not be confused with co-resident
kin. Indeed, a number of studies show that there are family members
available for most elders and maybe even increasingly so, in Sweden,
Britain, Belgium, and possibly other countries (Socialstyrelsen, 2004a;

Pickard et al., 2000; Audenaert, 2003). Often this is due to more elderly living into high age with a partner, frequently the most important and often also the most neglected family member.

Families Recover Ground in Sweden

In an analysis of care patterns, the elderly increasingly are *givers* of financial help and often provide as much care as they receive, in Sweden 24% and 21%, respectively (Socialstyrelsen, 2005). Data for Sweden, Norway, and other countries indicate substantial transfers from the elderly to children and grandchildren. Young, mostly single adults both in Southern and Northern Europe increasingly remain in (or return to) their parents' households, because of adverse labor and housing markets.

Most European elderly have children who live nearby and who often call, visit, or provide support and care. Indeed, as we have seen, Swedish families now help their elderly more than before. It is especially daughters who obey the commandment to honor one's parents: In 1994, 29% of the elderly (75+) were helped by female family members; in 2000, 39%. For those years, daughters made up 22% and 33%, respectively, of these figures. Help from males was constant at 15%, mostly from a son. (Daughters-in-law are less frequent in the panorama of care.) Usually, it is one person in the family who supports a frail elderly person: a spouse, a daughter, or a son. When a son is the main carer, often no daughter is available (Johansson, Sundström, & Hassing, 2003).

A recent survey gives some evidence about sentiments of filial responsibility and whether those sentiments can be actualized to support parents or not. A single question was used to explore this among middle-aged persons, shown in Table 3. The vast majority say that they can help, and more than one in ten already do.

Many may say that this trend increases the burden on the family. Yet, loosely referring to (burdens on) the family may be unfounded. Most elderly persons in Sweden have never cared for a parent (or anyone else), but if family care becomes more common–as it seems to be doing in Sweden–this will not necessarily mean a greater burden on the family but that more *family members* are helping their elders. Usually one person in the family provides the bulk of care. The interpretation of this development is complex and should avoid doctrinaire analytic schemes. Assessments should include how much these individual family members are doing and whether they stand alone with their commitment in their family and/or without public support. Regrettably, these predica-

TABLE 3. To Help Parents Is a Matter of Both Whether One Wants to and Whether One Can. Do You Have Any Possibility to Help and Support Your Parents or Do You Not? (by Age, Sweden 2001) (Percentages).

	Age	
	45-54	55-64
Help possibility, all		
Can help	63%	41%
Cannot help	8%	10%
Helping already today	10%	6%
No parents alive	17%	42%
Has parent(s) alive		
Can help	76%	72%
Cannot help	10%	18%
Helping already today	12%	10%

Source: Socialstyrelsen, 2004a.

ments often seem to be the case. In the Swedish case, there is often overlap between family and public services (Socialstyrelsen, 2004a; 2005); yet, the latter may be less than adequate. For a comparison, a small number of Spanish carers of dependent elders report that their cared-for persons also benefit from public services; many want these services to expand (IMSERSO, 2004).

Adult children can, as we have seen, help their parents–even more so today, as Table 4 shows. This derives from another survey that penetrated further the filial responsibility and to what extent various restrictions might hinder offspring from helping their parents. The survey was part of a government commission on the future availability of informal care.

One important conclusion that can be drawn from Tables 3 and 4 is that caring offspring can do more but that they do not want to stand alone with their commitment for frail parents, nor do the elderly want to be dependent solely on their offspring or other family. Both parties prefer a situation with some latitude of choice. Table 4 mirrors Swedish offsprings' attitudes to this. Another conclusion is that most offspring are unhindered by distance and even less by work from caring for parents. The majority can do more, especially if other family and/or the municipality share the commitment. Many (26%) already do what they

TABLE 4. To Help Parents Is a Matter of Both Whether One Wants to and Whether One Can, and What the Elders Themselves Prefer. Which of the Following Fits Your Situation? Persons 45+ with Parent(s) Alive, by Gender, Sweden 2002 (Several answers possible)

Helping Structure	All	Men	Women
Cannot do more due to distance	28%	22%	35%
Cannot do more due to work	9%	8%	10%
Can do more if the municipality takes a greater responsibility	11%	8%	14%
Can do more if other kin take a greater responsibility	3%	3%	4%
Can do more if both municipality and other kin take a greater responsibility	9%	8%	10%
Already doing much, cannot do more	22%	25%	20%
Already doing much, would like to cut down on what I do	4%	3%	4%
Don't know/no answer	29%	31%	26%

Source: Socialstyrelsen, 2004a.

can, whereof a minority (4%) would like to cut back on their commitments. The majority are in the 45-64 year age group.

The present and the desired division of responsibility between family and state is described by the offspring of frail elders in Table 5. The most common situation is one of *shared* responsibility, where the state bears the *main* responsibility. This is also the *desired* situation for persons who still have parents alive, whether their parents are frail and in need of help or not. The state cannot do everything, and people do not want it to. They want a fair balance of responsibility.

The concept of responsibility is somewhat evasive but "state main responsibility" doesn't necessarily mean that the state actually does most of the care, but *is* there, reliably and with quality care, in case needed. As mentioned, eventually 9 out of 10 elderly persons in Sweden will use public services. Many British and Swedish elderly say that they prefer professional care rather than family care, especially when they live alone and need intimate, long-term personal care. Similar results emerge from OASIS, a comparative study in Norway, England, Germany, Spain, and Israel. The majority of respondents, any age, want the responsibility to be shared. Few, anywhere, want the family *or* the state to be totally responsible for all old-age care (Daatland & Herlofson, 2003).

The greatest threat to a peaceful co-existence and collaboration in shared care–it might also be called solidarity–seems to be what was visible already in Table 2: the gradual focussing of public services primar-

TABLE 5. Actual and Desired Division of Responsibility Between Family and State (Municipality) for Frail Parents of Persons 45+ (Sweden 2002)

	Actual responsibility for frail parents	Desired responsibility for parent/s in case of need
State has full responsibility	34%	27%
State has main responsibility, family contributes	20%	48%
Family has main responsibility, state contributes	19%	15%
Family has full responsibility	29%	4%
No need for external help*	4%	2%
Other, don't know	3%	4%

* Typically, parents who help each other.
Source: Socialstyrelsen, 2004a.

ily on elders who lack immediate family and/or for some reason don't get cared for by family. The principle–common on the continent–that the state should intervene only in that situation is alien to modern Nordic welfare ideology, but Table 6 clearly shows that there is not only sharing of care, but also division of care: Elders who have spouses typically get very little public support. Those who have offspring get more, but the prime targets are elders without spouses or children. They are also the ones who to some extent rely on more distant kin and friends or neighbors. It is lucky, then, that elders increasingly have partners and children.

In recent surveys in the Nordic countries, adults, including the elderly, increasingly express dissatisfaction with the public services for the elderly and reveal distrust both in pensions and in public old-age care in the future. Yet, the general attitude in especially Northern Europe is to prefer public services to family or other providers, when needs are long-term. Partly popular discontent and distrust is rational; partly it is media-induced. Actual users of old-age care and their families are often happy with these services, but they can also express substantial dissatisfaction. It is possible that the problem in Swedish public services is one of quality rather than one of quantity. In Sweden as elsewhere, recruiting and retaining trained personnel is an ever growing problem. To complicate the picture further, there is also a good deal of "pluralistic ignorance": In surveys, many people still believe that the state is doing more and more and believe the family to do less and less.

TABLE 6. Support Patterns for Swedish Elders in Need of Help,* by Marital Status and Child Status, 2000, 75+. (Percentages).

	Has spouse/ partner		No spouse/ partner	
	Has offspring (N = 313)	No offspring (N = 37)	Has offspring (N = 320)	No offspring (N = 100)
Age (avg. years)	83%	82	86	86
% women	22	24	66	69
Help given only by				
Spouse/partner	70	70	-	-
Child(ren)**	3	3	30	-
Other kin	-	3	4	13
Other household member	-	-	2	-
Friend/neighbor	1	3	6	14
Home Help	5	3	21	34
Combinations of				
Spouse+child**	6	-	-	-
Spouse+Home Help	5	11	-	-
Spouse+other(s)	1	5	-	-
Child+HomeHelp**	1	-	19	-
Child+other(s)**	1	-	4	-
Home Help+other(s)	-	-	3	19
No one	6	5	12	19
Total	100	100	100	100

*Need help with one or more ADL-tasks
**Children include potential in-laws
Source: Computations on data for Hemma på äldre dar. Äldreuppdraget 2000:11, Socialstyrelsen 2000.

Policies and Support for Carers in Sweden

The 1998 amendment to the Social Service Act states that "the local authorities should support families and next of kin, when caring for elderly, sick and dependent family members." The law now carries a strong message to the municipalities to address support for carers. Further, in 1999, the Parliament launched a National Action Plan on Policy for the Elderly, including a renewed initiative to stimulate caregiver support (the "Carer-300 Project"). Between 1999-2001 a total of 300 million SEK (about 40 million U.S. dollars) of National grants were made available for the local authorities as an incentive to expand supportive services. Several steps have also been taken in recent years at the policy level.

Direct support to carers, added to the services provided to the elderly, in the modern sense was first established at a modest scale in the early 1950s, when scandalised authorities were unable to provide enough nursing home beds for the severely frail and sick. Old age homes in that era were filled with a mix of social cases and persons suffering from physical and/or mental deficiencies, which was in itself part of the scandals. The authorities then moved to provide a small financial allowance meant for carers, though paid to the patients (attendance allowance = hemsjukvårdsbidrag). It was soon followed by pro forma employment of family members as home helpers, culminating with some 19,000 recipients in 1970, who then made up a quarter of all home help personnel. For some municipalities this was primarily an inexpensive way to solve staffing shortages. The number of carers supported by these two programs has dwindled and is now some 7,100 persons altogether (2004). The reasons for this remain unclear, but it seems that many municipalities were uncomfortable with this hybrid, being neither family, nor professional. Also, it ran against the general principle in Swedish welfare primarily to provide services rather than cash.

Since 1989, there has also been the legal right, when a family member has a severe accident or illness and enters terminal care, for a worker to be on leave for up to 60 days (per cared for) with ordinary sick pay. This program, the Care Leave, is part of the National Social Insurance system. Annually, it is used by almost 10,000 people, mostly spouses and offspring.

The second type of support is respite care: both institutional and in-home respite care. In 1999, there were about 9,000 beds available for institutional respite care in Sweden. Another mode of respite care is adult day care. There are no data at the national level on how many day care units there are, but survey data from 1995 point to about 600 units in Sweden. In recent years, in-home respite, often free of charge, is offered in a growing number of municipalities.

The third type of support is counselling and personal support. In recent years, support groups have been very popular, usually run by voluntary organizations and now available all over the country. Counselling services in terms of a one-to-one contact is not provided on a regular basis.

In old age, care very much depends on the feeling of security. If public services can bolster this feeling, actual use of services may be low. Security is not to *use* a service, but to *get it*, reliably and swiftly, *when it is needed*. A few Swedish municipalities attempt to support carers by providing this kind of security through easy access to respite care. Without needs assessments or other bureaucratic hassle, an old person who uses public services may enter respite care any time that a perceived need arises. It is believed that this has lowered demand for residential care: People dare remain in their own homes and the actual use of respite care is relatively low. Many of these elders are at the receiving end of shared care.

The experiences and outcomes of the Carer-300 state grants were recently evaluated. A general experience is that it took a long time before local plans were implemented into action. Nevertheless, the number of support programs has steadily increased and municipalities have responded rapidly in expanding their supportive services for carers. However, we do not have any data on the quality of the programs, nor do we know how many carers they serve.

The development of carers' support has been spurred, and the result can be measured in quantitative terms and number of programs available. More critically, much of what has been done is not innovative, rather more of the same of familiar, old programs. At the same time, there is a growing "carers' movement" that continues to encourage national and local governments to provide easily accessible, flexible, and tailored support for carers.

To conclude, the carers' issue continues to stay on the social policy agenda in Sweden. In 2002, the Parliamentary Standing Committee on Health and Welfare commissioned the government to analyze the economic consequences of a new legislation on carer's right to service and support. The issue was to analyze the societal costs incurred if a defined group of carers (of all ages) would be provided with an undefined number of hours of in-home respite per week.

At the end of 2004, the Parliament decided not to proceed with improved legal rights to service and support. Instead, once again, the government is commissioned to elaborate promptly and present suggestions how service support for family carers can be improved and secured. New State grants to the municipalities were decided on for the period 2005-2007 to stimulate further development of support to carers.

CONCLUSION: CARE SHARED OR DIVIDED?

Solidarity seems to prevail in Sweden, expressed as preparedness to help or actual helping of needy elderly. In others words, solidarity between generations is not crowded out by an extensive public system of service and care for the elderly. Rather, it has recovered ground when public services have been curtailed in recent years. This is the main policy implication message of this article.

In Sweden, service provision has stagnated, and it is easy to find discontent among users and, especially, their families. Yet, decreasing coverage rates do not necessarily mean that the elderly are helped less often or that targeting is poorer today than before: More elders today may eventually use public services and end their lives in institutional care, and few elders are without public services before they die. For the welfare states these changes may, on average, imply a nearing to the continental pattern, where public services are less abundant. In the longer run, there may be a convergence of different welfare regimes, though the cultural tradition described at the outset probably continues to make a difference. Public old-age care in the Nordic countries has been comparatively successful in targeting needy elders. Few elders are lacking the help they need (Shea et al., 2003). This is due to a simple, one-stop administration, basically a heritage from the poor-relief era (above). Significant public responsibility for old-age care is a part of the Northern heritage, but its foundation is popular consent.

The cut in public service provision has also triggered a debate about "the societal contract" and whether the terms for the contract should be re-negotiated or not. In times of fewer public resources, cost containment, and a ceiling set on additional taxation, there is growing public debate about whether access to public service should be restricted in one way or the other.

Sweden seems to be heading towards a more mixed model of welfare provision, with a combination of public, informal, and market service provisions. However, families do not want to shoulder the *whole* burden of eldercare, nor do they want to abandon their elders. A *shared* commitment may be the modern meaning of solidarity. Although sharing of care between family and state took place already in pre-welfare times in the Nordic countries, it certainly has grown in scope. A gloomy scenario for this kind of solidarity between caring families and the state is the tendency for public services to *divide* care, by primarily focussing on elders who have little family care at the risk of neglecting those with more abundant family support.

What has happened in recent years, at least in Sweden and probably elsewhere as well, is the dislocation of the balance between families and state. Families are doing more than before for their elders. This, one would expect, should call forth *more* support for carers, rather than less. In the interface between informal and formal care, there are two vital and interconnected issues for the Swedish model. The first issue has to do with the problems of safeguarding the level of present public services and care in Sweden. This concerns the legitimacy of the system of welfare for older people in our country. A second issue is whether the formal services are able to respond to the needs and demands of the caregivers. The challenge, then, is to strike a balance in optimizing family and public resources, in a partnership of care.

AUTHOR NOTES

Lennarth Johansson, Psychologist, Associate Professor of Gerontology, has over 20 years' experiences as Senior Researcher, specialized in housing, services, and care for the elderly. His main interest is informal care and social policy aspects of elderly care. Since 1993 he has been research leader at the National Board of Health and Welfare, responsible for national follow-up and evaluation of recent reforms in care for the elderly in Sweden. Professor Johansson can be contacted at Socialstyrelsen, S-106 30 Stockholm, Sweden (E-mail: lennarth.johansson@socialstyrelsen.se).

Gerdt Sundström, Sociologist and Professor of Gerontology, has worked at the Institute of Gerontology in Jönköping since 1985. His main interests are services for the elderly, especially Home Help, and patterns of family care, in Sweden and internationally. He has researched and published widely on these subjects. Professor Sundström can be contacted at Institute of Gerontology, School of Health Sciences, Box 1026, S-551 11 Jönköping, Sweden (E-mail: gerdt.sundstrom@hhj.hj.se).

The authors thank two anonymous reviewers for their valuable comments.

REFERENCES

Audenaert, V. (2003). Changes in older people's living arrangements in Flanders, 1993-98. *Ageing & Society, 23(*4): 451-470.

Bengtson, V. L., & Roberts, R. E. L. (1991). Intergenerational solidarity in aging families: An example of formal theory construction. *Journal of Marriage and the Family, 53*: 856-870.

Daatland, S. O., & Herlofson, K. (2003). 'Lost solidarity' or 'changed solidarity': A comparative European view of normative family solidarity. *Ageing & Society, 23(*5): 537-560.

Glaser, K., Hancock, R., & Stuchbury, R. (1998). Attitudes in an ageing society. Research sponsored by Age Concern England for the Millennium Debate of the Age, Age Concern Institute of Gerontology, London.

Glaser, K., & Tomassini, C. (2003). Demography: Living arrangements, receipt of care, residential proximity and housing preferences among older people in Britain and Italy in the 1990s: An overview of trends. In Sumner, K. (Ed.) *Our homes, our lives: Choice in later life living arrangements.* London: Centre for Policy on Ageing.

IMSERSO (Instituto de Mayores y Servicios Sociales) (2004). Apoyo Informal. Documentos technicos. www.mtas.es/imsermo

Johansson, L., Sundström, G., & Hassing, L. B. (2003). State Down, Off-Spring Up: The Substitution Issue in Old-Age Care Reversed in Sweden. *Ageing & Society,* 23(3): 269-280.

Lingsom, S. (1997). The Substitution Issue. Oslo, NOVA, Rapport 6/97.

Millar, J., & Warman, H. (1996). *Family Obligations in Europe.* London: Family Policy Studies Centre.

Pickard, L. et al. (2000). Relying on informal care in the new century? Informal care for elderly people in England to 2031. *Ageing and Society,* 20(6): 745-772.

Platz, M. (1989). Gamle i eget hjem. Bind 1: Levekår. Socialforskningsinstituttet, Rapport 89:12.

Senior (2005). Äldrepolitik för framtiden: SOU 2003:91 (Old Age Policy for the Future, government white paper).

Shanas, E. et al. (1968). Old People in Three Industrial Societies. London: Routledge & Kegan Paul.

Shea, D., Davey, A., Femia, E., Zarit, S., Sundström, G., Berg, S., & Smyer, A. (2003). Exploring assistance in Sweden and the United States. *The Gerontologist,* 43(5): 712-721.

Skoglund, A-M. (1992). Fattigvården på den svenska landsbygden år 1829 (Poor relief in Sweden 1829). School of Social Work, University of Stockholm, *Rapport i socialt arbete 58.* Diss.

Socialstyrelsen (2004a). Framtidens anhörigomsorg (Future availability of infomal care). (*www.sos.se)* (authors Lennarth Johansson & Gerdt Sundström).

Socialstyrelsen (2004b). Äldres levnadsförhållanden 1988-2002 (Living conditions of Elderly 1988-2002). (*www.sos.se)* (authors Bo Malmberg & Gerdt Sundström)

Socialstyrelsen (2005). Likhet inför äldreomsorgen (Equity in old age care in Sweden? Municipal variations and the Family). (*www.sos.se)* (authors Bo Malmberg & Gerdt Sundström)

SOU (1956). Åldringsvård (Old Age Care, government white paper).

Sundström, G. (1983). *Caring for the Aged in Welfare Society.* School of Social Work, University of Stockholm *Stockholm Studies in Social Work 1.* Diss.

Sundström, G. (1994). Care by Families: An Overview of Trends, in *Caring for Frail Elderly People. New Directions in Care.* Paris, OECD, Social Policy Studies No. 14.

Sundström, G. (1999). Social policy and life-styles of the elderly in the Scandinavian countries and in France. In *Comparing Social Welfare Systems in Nordic Europe and France.* Copenhagen Conference. Volume 4. CNRS & Ministère de l'Emploi et de la Solidarité. Paris.

Sundström, G. et al. (2003). Informal Care in the North and South of Europe. A Comparative Analysis. Presentation at Vth European Congress of Gerontology, Barcelona, July 2-5, 2003 (in collaboration with Lars Andersson, Karen Glaser, Emily Grundy, Maria Iacovou, Mayte Sancho Castiello and Cecilia Tomassini).

Sundström, G., Johansson, L., & Hassing, L. (2002). The shifting balance of long-term care in Sweden. *The Gerontologist*, *42*(3): 350-355.

Sundström, G., Johansson, L., Malmberg, B., Romören, T. I., & Samuelsson, G. (2003). Innan döden skiljer oss åt. (Before Death Does Us Apart). *Aldring & Livslöp*, *1*: 24-29.

Tomassini, C., Wolf, D., & Rosina, A. (2003). Parental Housing Assistance and Parent-Child Proximity in Italy. *Journal of Marriage and Family*, *65*: 700-715.

Tornstam, L. (2005). Personal communication.

doi:10.1300/J031v18n03_02

Danish Home Care Policy and the Family: Implications for the United States

Mary Stuart, ScD

University of Maryland Baltimore County

Eigil Boll Hansen, MSc

Institute of Local Government Studies, Copenhagen, Denmark

SUMMARY. This paper provides an overview of reforms in Danish long-term care initiated in the early 1980s, describes the relationship between elder care in Denmark and the family, and considers implications for U.S. policy. The success of Denmark's community-based experimentation with new models of home care and housing for the elderly resulted in a national decision to eliminate new construction of nursing homes and increase access to publicly funded home care. Lingering concern that the provision of paid assistance for the elderly could undermine family structure is allayed by the findings of a recent survey: Three-fourths of the elderly report seeing their children on a weekly or more frequent basis. Findings from the Danish experience provide evidence that community-based services can aid family caregivers, enable the frail elderly to live in the setting of their choice, and be cost-effective from a public policy perspective. doi:10.1300/J031v18n03_03 *[Article copies available for a fee from The Haworth Document Delivery Service: 1-800-HAWORTH. E-mail address: <docdelivery@haworthpress.com> Website:*

[Haworth co-indexing entry note]: "Danish Home Care Policy and the Family: Implications for the United States." Stuart, Mary, and Eigil Boll Hansen. Co-published simultaneously in *Journal of Aging & Social Policy* (The Haworth Press, Inc.) Vol. 18, No. 3/4, 2006, pp. 27-42; and: *Family and Aging Policy* (ed: Francis G. Caro) The Haworth Press, Inc., 2006, pp. 27-42. Single or multiple copies of this article are available for a fee from The Haworth Document Delivery Service [1-800-HAWORTH, 9:00 a.m. - 5:00 p.m. (EST). E-mail address: docdelivery@haworthpress.com].

KEYWORDS. Danish elder care, home care policy, community-based care, paid assistance

INTRODUCTION

Denmark has been widely recognized as a country that has implemented cost-effective community-based systems of home care for the frail elderly. In the early 1980s, with a high proportion of women in the labor force and a growing population of elderly citizens, Denmark initiated a process of reforming an institutional system of long-term care. Today, extensive service networks that integrate health, home care, and personal care can be found in nearly all of Denmark's 271 local municipalities. What impact does this system have on family relations and family care-giving? In this paper we review the basics of Danish long-term care and discuss how public services and families interact in providing assistance to the frail elderly. We then consider the implications for U.S. policy as this country seeks to meet the growing need for services for the old elderly.

OVERVIEW OF DANISH SOCIAL POLICY

To understand the Danish system of providing services for elders who need assistance with activities of daily living (ADLs), an overview of the basic principles of Danish social policy and a brief description of the developments in elder care during the last 20 years are useful. In contrast to the United States, five fundamental principles of health and social services apply to the care for older people: (1) Services are financed largely by general taxes, rather than user payment and private contributions. They are available largely without charge to consumers. (2) Service coverage is universal. All citizens are entitled to the services, and eligibility is based on an assessment of the needs of the individual and his or her household. (3) Responsibility for health and social services are decentralized to local counties and municipalities. Denmark has 271 local jurisdictions, known as municipalities, which range in size from 2,300 to 496,000 inhabitants. Municipal services (including personal care, home health care, nursing homes, and primary medical care) are financed through local income and property taxes as well as block grants from the central government. (4) National policy and regulations for elder care are established by the Danish Parliament and the central government. (5) Services are generally provided by the local government rather than by private or voluntary organizations. In January 2003, a new policy directed that recipients of home help should have the option of choosing a private provider for assistance financed by the local government. However, not all municipalities have a private provider, and less than 10% of the recipients of home help have chosen a private provider (Ankestyrelsen, 2004).

BUILDING BLOCKS IN DANISH ELDER POLICY

The foundation of the contemporary Danish system of elder care dates to around 1980. At that time a national Commission on Aging completed a report, formulating principles for future policies on care and housing for older people in Denmark. One of the key recommendations was that long-term care policy should be better organized to compensate for losses that occur with aging. The Commission advocated policies and practices that would support the potential for older adults with disabilities to continue living active and independent lives, preserve self determination, and facilitate continuity in their housing. In particular, the Commission recommended that arrangements for housing and support services for older dependent people should be organized so that they do not have to move as the need for help increases. The Commission advised that services be developed that would enable the municipalities gradually to increase help as needed in the older person's home (or in a dwelling where he or she had chosen to move).

At approximately the same time, several municipalities introduced 24-hour home-care systems. Other developments of significance followed, most notably an increase in special dwellings that were adapted to provide handicapped accessibility (and in some cases, staff) and where the residents are considered as tenants (rather than patients), a decline in nursing home beds, and an increase in the number and percentage of the elderly receiving home help from municipalities. A brief history and description of these pivotal developments follows. For a more extensive discussion of the development of the Danish system, see Stuart and Weinrich, 2001a and 2001b, among other sources.

Twenty-Four Hour Integrated Home Care

During the 1980s several municipalities experimented with the 24-hour/7-day per week home-care system. For evening and night shifts, personal care providers and home health nurses used a car and a wireless radio connected to a common staffed base. Elderly people needing urgent assistance could call a central number for help using the phone or an alarm system (such as those worn on wrist bands). This system made it possible to respond quickly and efficiently to the care needs of fragile elderly who were living in the community. Additional efficiency was obtained by municipalities through the *integrated care system,* in which staff from the local nursing home and home care organization were combined into a single organization to care for the frail elderly in a geographic area. With this system, the same staff could provide assistance to people living in ordinary housing, adapted special dwellings, and nursing homes. This arrangement offered flexibility; the municipality gave personal care and nursing services based on the needs of the citizen, irrespective of the type of housing. Piloted initially in Skaevinge under the direction of Lis Wagner, RN (Wagner, 1997), today almost all Danish municipalities have 24-hour integrated home-care systems (Stuart and Weinrich, 2001a and 2001b).

Housing for Older People

During the 1980s, municipalities also began to experiment with new types of dwellings for dependent older people as a substitute for nursing homes. The most common type of new housing had adaptations to meet the needs of older people with physical disabilities. Usually housing units were congregate, sometimes with staff, social activities, exercise equipment, or rehabilitation facilities. A typical housing unit consisted of two rooms, and a kitchen and a bathroom. The dwellings were serviced by the 24-hour home-care system. This remains the prototype of dwellings for dependent older people in Denmark (Hansen, 2002). Admittance to special dwellings is granted by the local authority of a municipality and depends on an assessment of the applicant's disabilities and the possibility of receiving adequate help in his or her ordinary dwelling. Special dwellings are not institutions, and residents are similar to tenants.

In 1988, legislation was implemented that prohibited municipalities from building nursing homes. The effect of policies that encouraged construction of assisted living units and prohibited nursing home construction resulted in a dramatic increase in adapted special dwellings between 1985 and 1999 (3,207 to 32,501) and a reduction in nursing homes (49,487 to 31,244). Approximately one-third of the adapted special dwellings have 24-hour staffing. Staffed housing is generally reserved for individuals with severe dementia or those who require high levels of supervision (Hansen, 2002).

A 1995 survey (Hansen & Platz, 1995a) found that about 50% of people defined as "physically vulnerable" aged 80+ lived in ordinary dwellings or adapted dwellings cared for by the home-care system. Half of these people lived alone. People were considered "physically vulnerable" if they were not able to walk out of doors and thought they had poor health; if they needed help getting in and out of bed, washing/bathing, dressing, or using the toilet.

Home Help and Other Home Care Services

Home help, including assistance with domestic tasks such as housecleaning and personal care such as dressing and bathing, is another of the basic services that municipalities provide for the frail elderly free of charge. Home help is granted on the basis of an assessment of the household's ability to take care of various types of housework and personal care. Typically, home help personnel of the municipal provider are part of a multidisciplinary team that includes a nurse. Individuals providing these services are required to have completed a specific educational program of at least one year (Hansen & Platz, 1995a).

Other home care services provided by the municipality include home nursing, which is generally short-term and prescribed by a physician to provide specified prevention or treatment. In addition, municipalities typically offer day care, night care, respite care, acute care, and rehabilitation services for the frail elderly who live at home (Hansen & Platz, 1995b). Most municipalities provide transportation for health and social activities for the elderly. In many municipalities, day centers provide rehabilitation and maintenance physical therapy and occupational therapy to promote functioning and prevent deterioration. The majority of municipalities also have specialized housing for individuals with dementia (Hansen & Platz, 1995b).

Attitudes Towards the Responsibility for Assistance

Only 3% of elders aged 70 or older in Denmark live with their children (Kahler, 1992). However, the Danish policy analysts assert that

Danish social legislation is based on the premise that citizens bear the primary responsibility for themselves and their families. For older people, this essentially means in practice that in addition to the responsibility for themselves, spouses also have a mutual responsibility for each other. If an elderly person in need of care lives in a household with an adult child, the child will have to contribute to the housekeeping, but not necessarily fulfill needs for personal care. Legislation puts no obligations on children or other family members not living in the same household to care for dependent elders.

A recent Danish study (Colmorten et al., 2003) concludes that the principle that one should be responsible for taking care of oneself reflects the attitudes of older people, relatives, and other parties such as municipal employees, local politicians, and volunteer and special interest organizations. If an elderly person in need of assistance has a spouse, the general attitude is that the spouse should help. Assistance from the public sector is expected only when the household is unable to take care of the housekeeping or personal care itself. However, a majority of older people think that older people who can clean their houses only with great difficulty also have the right to receive public home help.

In the study, the older people of the survey and relatives in focus groups were asked to consider who should provide assistance with different types of task. The answers can be summed up as follows:

- With regard to domestic tasks, they are primarily the responsibility of the spouse. The municipality should provide assistance only when an older couple is not able to handle such tasks themselves and in cases where there is no spouse. Assistance paid for privately and help from family and friends or neighbors play only minor roles in this context.
- With regard to dealing with the authorities and with money matters, it is also primarily the spouse's responsibility, and if there is no spouse who can take care of these matters, then it is, first and foremost, the family who should take on such responsibilities. The municipality is attributed only a small amount of responsibility, and that is only for single older people.
- With regard to getting out of doors, it is primarily the responsibility of the spouse, followed by the municipality, according to older people and their relatives. The family is attributed more responsibility with regard to older people without spouses as opposed to older couples. Volunteer organizations are not mentioned very of-

ten by older people, while relatives think that such organizations could play greater roles.

- With regard to the need for a more suitable residence, it is primarily the municipality's responsibility, followed by the individual older person, and finally by the family.
- With regard to the need to participate in leisure-time activities or the need for someone to talk to, the older person is primarily responsible, while the municipality is not attributed any degree of responsibility worth mentioning except in cases involving older people with no spouse and with greatly reduced functional capacity (Colmorten et al., 2003, p. 104).

Assistance to Older People

There have been several studies on assistance to older people with various types of housework and they all show the same tendencies. Table 1 reports findings from a survey conducted in 2002.

Households with older people *mostly* take care of the housework themselves, and except for what is defined as difficult cleaning, less than 5% of households with people below age 82 have others to do most of the housework tasks. If older people do not mostly themselves take

TABLE 1. People Aged 67, 72, 77, or 82 in 2002 Distributed According to Who *Mostly* Takes Care of Various Types of Housework (Percentages) (Excluding People in Nursing Homes)

	Difficult cleaning[1]	Easier cleaning[2]	Shopping	Washing clothes	Hot meal
Household	78	96	92	95	93
Home help (e.g., municipality)	14	2	1	3	0
Family, friends, other	2	1	6	2	1
Assistance paid for	6	1	1	1	0
Meals-on-wheels	•	•	•	•	3
Eat out	•	•	•	•	2
Do not usually eat hot meal	•	•	•	•	0
In total	100	100	100	101	99
Number of cases	*3,346*	*3,355*	*3,346*	*3,351*	*3,363*

[1] For example, vacuum-cleaning, washing the floor, washing stairs.
[2] For example, dusting, tidying up.
• = Irrelevant
Source: Special analysis on The Danish Longitudinal Database on Aging. Data are from a survey in 2002 among a representative sample of people in Denmark born in 1920, 1925, 1930, 1935, 1940, 1945, or 1950. The total number of respondents is 8,207 (response rate 81).

care of difficult cleaning, the public home help does, and in just a few cases family or friends mostly take care of difficult cleaning. Family and friends play a role by shopping regularly and to a lesser extent by washing clothes regularly. If older people do not prepare hot meals themselves, they usually receive meals-on-wheels or eat out in a center or in a restaurant.

Few older people pay for having the housework done. Those who do may not be eligible for publicly financed home help, or they may be unsatisfied with the quality of the help they can get from the home help system.

The ranking of the resources of help is the same for people aged 80 and above, but in this age group the households themselves take care of fewer tasks (Table 2).

This analysis is based on questions, including "Who mostly takes care of?" Family and friends could provide assistance with cleaning, shopping, washing clothes, etc., without doing it "mostly." In 2002, the sample population was asked whether within the latest month they had received help from family or friends with, for example, housework. Table 3 shows the share that confirmed they had received help.

It is not possible to state exactly what help older people have received from family or friends, but one can conclude that it is not common for

TABLE 2. People Aged 80+ in 1994 Distributed According to Who *Mostly* Takes Care of Various Types of Housework (Percentages) (Excluding People in Nursing Homes)

	Cleaning[1]	Shopping	Washing clothes	Hot meal
Household	40	60	60	70
Children or other family	3	12	10	3
Home help	51	21	21	1
Others	6	7	8	2
Meals-on-wheels	•	•	•	19
Eat out	•	•	•	5
Do not usually eat hot meal	•	•	•	0
In total	100	100	99	100
Number of cases	*1,683*	*1,683*	*1,683*	*1,683*

[1] In this case it is not possible to distinguish between difficult and easier cleaning.
• = Irrelevant
Source: (Hansen et al., 2002). Data are from a survey in 1994 among a representative sample of people aged 80+ in 75 Danish municipalities. The total number of respondents is 1,845 (response rate 78).

older people in Denmark to receive help with housework from family or friends. The most common help is with maintaining the house or gardening, although only 13% of all the persons in the age group have received such help within the latest month (The Danish Longitudinal Database on Aging).

In Table 3, the share of older people having received help from family or friends is considerably higher than in Table 1. This can be explained by the fact that Table 3 includes more occasionally provided help, while Table 1 includes only help provided on a regular basis. Furthermore, the people included in Table 3 are on average more dependent on help than the people included in Table 1.

Studies on care for older people have not included help with personal chores such as bathing, dressing, and getting in and out of bed. This may be based on the assumption that spouses may help each other in case of disablement. In case of disabled people living alone, help with personal chores is provided by the public home-care system, while help from children or other family members is very rare. Lewinter (Lewinter, 1999) states that personal care is the task of the home help because this formalized intimacy is easier to handle for both older people and their families, and it supports the preserving of older people's feeling of integrity as taboo fields have not been crossed.

Social Contacts

Table 4 shows figures for how often older people in Denmark see their children. Very few older people in Denmark live with one or more of their children, but the great majority of older people usually see (one of) their children once a week, the oldest not quite as often as those in their seventies.

TABLE 3. The Share of People Aged 67, 72, 77, or 82 in 2002 Who Had Received Help from Family or Friends with Housework Within the Latest Month (Percentages) (Excluding People in Nursing Homes)

	Have received help	Number of cases
People having difficulties in doing difficult cleaning or cannot do it	22	961
People having difficulties in shopping or cannot do it	25	663
People having difficulties in washing clothes or cannot do it	25	476

Source: Special analysis on The Danish Longitudinal Database on Aging. See Table 1.

It is also evident from the preceding figures that despite not having the primary responsibility to provide housecleaning and personal care for the frail elderly, Danish children still visit their aging parents regularly. Do they do so more or less than children in other countries? A comparative study on selected European countries found that older people in Denmark were more likely than those in Germany to meet relatives or friends often, while the share is less when Denmark is compared with Greece, Holland, and England. There is no significant difference between Denmark and Italy on this indicator (Arendt et al., 2003). There is no clear evidence from this study that older people in Denmark have weaker or stronger social relations than older people in other countries.

DISCUSSION

Much has been written regarding the effects that race and ethnic and cultural differences play in the experiences of family caregivers within the United States (Dilworth-Anderson, 2002). The potential for ethnic and cultural differences is magnified when making comparisons between countries. Given the long-standing differences between Denmark and the United States in attitudes regarding the importance of a public "safety-net," we must be cautious in generalizing from the results of Danish social policy for the United States. It is, however, because of the substantial differences in U.S. and Danish long-term care policies that

TABLE 4. People Aged 72 or 77 in 1997 and People Aged 80+ in 1995 and Having Living Children Distributed According to When They Last Saw (One of) Their Children (Percentages) (Excluding People in Nursing Homes)

When did you last see (one of) your children?	People aged 72 or 77		People aged 80+	
	Men	Women	Men	Women
Live with child	4	2	5	4
Today or yesterday	38	37	33	37
2-7 days ago	35	43	35	34
8-30 days ago	16	12	19	18
More than a month ago	6	6	8	7
In total	*99*	*100*	*100*	*100*
Number of cases	*707*	*1,273*	*504*	*885*

Source: (Platz, 2000) and (Hansen & Platz, 1996). Data on people aged 72 or 77 are from a survey in 1997 among a representative sample of people in Denmark born in 1920, 1925, 1930, 1935, 1940, or 1945. The total number of respondents is 5,864 (response rate 70). Data on people aged 80+, see Table 2.

the Danish experiment is worth closer examination by U.S. policy-makers.

Table 5 enumerates some of the statistics that highlight major structural differences between the Danish and U.S. approaches to long-term care. Most notably, Denmark has a higher percentage of women in the labor force when compared to the United States (73% vs. 59%); half the number of nursing home beds per 1,000 people 65+ (26 vs. 52); and a far higher percentage of elderly receiving home help (49% of people 80+ vs. 5%).

When the frail elderly in Denmark require home help, these services are generally provided without charge by the local municipality. By contrast, when home health care is purchased in the United States, 36% is paid for out of private funds (NHES, 2004).

The amount of housekeeping and personal care services provided by family members for the frail elderly, as well as the level of out-of-pocket payments for long-term care services, are very different between the two countries. Only a small percentage of the frail elderly in Denmark lives with their families or receives help with housecleaning and

TABLE 5. Comparative Statistics on Denmark and the United States

	Denmark[a] 2004	United States 2004
Total population	5.4 million	294 million
Percentage aged 65+	15%	12%[b]
Percentage aged 80+	4%	4%[b]
Percentage women in the labour force	73%[1]	59%[2,c]
Nursing home places per 1,000 65+	26	52[d]
Nursing home places per 1,000 80+	97	180[d]
Percentage of 65+ receiving home help	22%	3%[e]
Percentage of 80+ receiving home help	49%	5%[e]

[1]Age 16-66
[2]Age 16+
Sources:
[a]Statistics Denmark: www.statistikbanken.dk
[b]U.S. Census Bureau: http://www.census.gov/popest/national/asrh/NC-EST2004-sa.html
[c]Bureau of Labor Statistics: Women in the Labor Force: A Databook: www.bls.gov/cps/wlfdata book200r.htm
[d]National Center for Health Statistics: National Nursing Home Survey 1999: http://www.cdc.gov/nchs/data/nnhsd/NNHS99selectedchar_homes_beds_residents.pdf
[e]National Center for Health Statistics: Current Home Health Care Patients 2000: http://www.cdc.gov/nchs/data/nhhcsd/curhomecare00.pdf

personal care on a regular basis from family members outside their household. By contrast, in America, "the voluminous body of research concerning the long-term caregiving needs of frail elders . . . suggests one principal conclusion: Families are their primary and most effective source of support. Family members provide 60-80% of long-term care for dependent elderly members, and formal or institutional mechanisms become activated only after family caregiving resources are expended. This is documented in extensive research reviews" (Bengtson, Rosenthal et al., 1996).

A major barrier to increasing community-based services for the elderly in the United States has been the concern that doing so would result in increases in public expenditures. However, the opposite has occurred in Denmark. During the 12-year period from 1985 to 1997, long-term care expenditures (including durable medical supplies, equipment, and nursing home expenditures for the non-elderly disabled as well as the elderly populations) for the over-80 population in the United States increased a whopping 68%, while comparable per capita expenditures in Denmark decreased 12% and declined as a percentage of gross domestic product (Stuart & Weinrich, 2001a). While per capita long-term care expenditures for the population 80+ were considerably higher in Denmark than in the United States in 1985, by 1997 those expenditures were approximately the same in both countries (Stuart & Weinrich, 2001a). While the average per capita costs may be roughly the same in both countries, the distribution of expenditures differs enormously. In the United States, expenditures are concentrated on a relatively small number of people who receive care in high-cost institutional settings. Conversely, the Danes are spending their resources on home care, where they serve far more people at a lower cost per person served.

Economic analysis of municipal variation in Denmark suggests that services for the frail elderly are more efficient when the reliance on nursing homes is low, relative to home care services (Hansen, 1998). Thus, the need for efficiency in providing health and social services combined with a commitment to enabling people to remain in the community have led the Danes to maximize the development of efficient public home care services. Denmark has the highest level of home care among the European countries, providing nearly two times the hours of home help for the elderly as Sweden, the next closest country for this indicator (Danish Government, 2000).

What is the impact of this responsibility on families? While some research has emphasized the positive benefits of intergenerational caring, including the reciprocal role that elders can play in families (Lopata,

1993), reciprocity declines as the parent's health deteriorates (Spitz, 1992). Depression, burden, role strain, relationship strain, and psychological distress have all been identified as negative effects associated with family caregiving. Dilworth-Anderson, Williams et al., and Lawton, Rajagopal et al. found that greater burden was directly associated with greater depression (Dilworth-Anderson, Williams et al., 2002; Lawton, Rajagopal et al., 1992). High levels of relationship strain have been reported using a composite measure that includes the "caregiver's feelings of being pressured, angry, depressed, manipulated, strained, resentful, depended upon, and the feeling that the relationship had a negative effect on other family members" (Cox, 1993). Another study found that nearly one-third of caregivers reported that their health had deteriorated as a result of caregiving (Cox & Monk, 1993). A recent study found that caregivers who experienced caregiver strain had mortality risks that were 63% higher than non-caregiving controls (Schulz & Beach, 1999). Stress has been identified as a risk factor for elder abuse in the United States (Pillemer & Suitor, 1992). "The most pervasive consequence of caregiving is the emotional strain generated by the burdens placed on the caregiver . . . Competing demands, and childrearing and employment in particular, have been considered potential sources of stress" (Stone, Cafferata et al., 1987).

When there is no spouse to provide assistance, the caregiving role falls primarily to daughters and daughters-in-laws in the United States (Horowitz, 1985). In contrast to studies in Denmark, Brody and colleagues found that housework and laundry are among the activities that daughters frequently provided, regardless of their employment status, and when these services are obtained from outside sources, they were generally privately paid for rather than subsidized by the government (Brody & Schoonover, 1986).

CONCLUSION

As the United States faces continuing increases in long-term care costs, a growing percentage of old elderly, increases in life expectancy, and a high percentage of women in the labor force, the efficiency of the Danish municipal service systems should be attractive to U.S. policymakers. If the United States could import such a system, would it be good for families? There is evidence that social supports can mitigate the negative effects of caregiving stressors (Pearlin, Aneshensel et al., 1996). There is also evidence that the types of assistance that elderly women are most willing to receive from non-family members are personal care and household help (Brody, Johnsen et al., 1984), two of the services the elderly are most likely to receive from the municipalities in Denmark. This same study (Brody, Johnsen et al., 1984) found that the types of supports the elderly preferred to receive from their children included emotional support and financial management–supports frequently provided by families in Denmark as well.

Some would argue that taking away the responsibility of caring for elderly people from the family would weaken elderly people's family network. The Danish case brings no support to this argument, since elderly people's contact with their children is just as frequent in Denmark as in other European countries with more obligations on the family. The family is still involved in practical, social, and emotional dimensions of the care for elderly people (Lewinter, 1999), but the burden of caring–or at least some of it–is relieved through public assistance.

AUTHOR NOTES

Mary Stuart, ScD, is Professor and Director, Health Administration and Policy Program, University of Maryland Baltimore County (UMBC). She ws formerly Director of Policy for the Maryland Department of Health and Mental Hygiene. Dr. Stuart can be reached at the University of Maryland Baltimore County (UMBC), 1000 Hilltop Circle, Baltimore, MD 21250 (E-mail: stuart@umbc.edu).

Eigil Boll Hansen, MSc, is Associate Professor of Economics at Amternes og Kommunernes Forskningsinstitut (AKF), Institute of Local Government Studies, Copenhagen, Denmark. Mr. Hansen can be contacted at AKF, Nyropsgade 37, 1602 Copenhagen, Denmark (E-mail: ebh@akf.dk).

REFERENCES

Ankestyrelsen (2004). *Frit valg i aeldreplejen–erfaringer fra landets kommuner.* Copenhagen: Ankestyrelsen.

Arendt, J. N., Hansen, E. B., Olsen, H., Rasmussen, M., Bentzen, J., & Rimdal, B. (2003). *Levevilkaar blandt folkepensionister uden supplerende indkomst. 03*:15. Copenhagen: Socialforskningsinstituttet.

Bengtson, V., Rosenthal, C. et al. (1996). Paradoxes of Families and Aging, in *Handbook of Aging and the Social Sciences*, L. George and R. Binstock (Eds.). San Diego: Academic Press: 255.

Brody, E. M., Johnsen, P. T. et al. (1984). What should adult children do for elderly parents? Opinions and preferences of three generations of women. *J Gerontol, 39*(6): 736-46.

Brody, E. M., & Schoonover, C. B. (1986). Patterns of parent-care when adult daughters work and when they do not. *Gerontologist, 26*(4): 372-81.

Colmorten, E., Hansen, E. B., Pedersen, S., Platz, M., & Roenow, B. (2003). Den aeldre har brug for hjaelp. Hvem boer traede til? Copenhagen: AKF Forlaget.

Cox, C. (1993). Service needs and interests: A comparison of African American and White caregivers seeking Alzheimer's assistance. *American Journal of Alzheimer's Care and Related Disorders and Research, 8*(3): 35.

Cox, C., & Monk, A. (1993). Hispanic culture and family care of Alzheimer's patients. *Health Soc Work, 18*(2): 92-100.

Danish Government, The (2000). Structural Monitoring–International Benchmarking of Denmark. Copenhagen: The Ministry of Finance.

Dilworth-Anderson, P., Williams, I. C. et al. (2002). Issues of race, ethnicity, and culture in caregiving research: A 20-year review (1980-2000). *Gerontologist, 42*(2): 237-72.

Hansen, E. B. (1998). Social Protection for Dependency in Old Age in Denmark.in Department of Health. Modernising and Improving EU Social Protection: Conference on Long-Term Care of Elderly Dependent People in the EU and Norway. London: Department of Health Publications.

Hansen, E. B. (2002). Häusliche Versorgung fur Hilfebedürftige und Schwerkranke in Dänemark. in D. Schaeffer/M. Ewers (Eds.). *Ambulant vor stationär. Perspektiven für eine integrierte ambulante Pflege Schwerkranker.* Gottingen, Verlag Hans Huber.

Hansen, E. B., Milkaer, L., Swane, C. E., Iversen, C. L., & Rimdal, B. (2002). Mange Baekke smaa...om hjaelp til svaekkede aeldre. Copenhagen: FOKUS.

Hansen, E. B., & Platz, M. (1995). 80-100-åriges levekaar. Copenhagen: AKF Forlaget.

Hansen, E. B., & Platz, M. (1995b). Kommunernes tilbud til aeldre. Copenhagen: AKF Forlaget.

Hansen, E. B., & Platz, M. (1996). Gamle danskere. Copenhagen: AKF Forlaget.

Horowitz, A. (1985). Family caregiving to the frail elderly. *Annu Rev Gerontol Geriatr, 5*: 194-246.

Kahler, M. (1992). Ten years after the Commission on Aging–ideas and results. *Danish Medical Bulletin, 39*: 216-219.

Lawton, M. P., Rajagopal, D. et al. (1992). The dynamics of caregiving for a demented elder among black and white families. *J Gerontol, 47*(4): S156-64.

Lewinter, M. (1999). Spreading the burden of gratitude-elderly between family and state. Copenhagen: Sociologisk Institut.

Lopata, H. Z. (1993). The interweave of public and private: Women's challenge to American society. *Journal of Marriage and the Family, 55*: 176-190.

NHES (2004). National health care expenditures projections tables. Table 10, Centers for Medicare and Medicaid Services.

Pearlin, L., Aneshensel, C. et al. (1996). Caregiving and its social support, in *Handbook of Aging and the Social Sciences*, L. George and R. Binstock (Eds.). San Diego: Academic Press: 283-302.

Pillemer, K. & Suitor, J. J. (1992). Violence and violent feelings: What causes them among family caregivers? *J Gerontol, 47*(4): S165-72.

Platz, M. (2000). Danskere med livserfaring–portraetteret i tal. Copenhagen: Socialforskningsinstituttet.

Schulz, R., & Beach, S. R. (1999). Caregiving as a risk factor for mortality: The Caregiver Health Effects Study. *Jama, 282*(23): 2215-19.

Spitz, G., &. Logan, J. (1992). Helping as a component of parent-child relations. *Research on Aging, 14*(3): 291-312.

Stone, R., Cafferata, G. et al. (1987). Caregivers of the Frail Elderly: A National Profile. *The Gerontologist, 27*(5): 616-626.

Stuart, M., & Weinrich, M. (2001a). Home- and community-based long-term care: Lessons from Denmark. *Gerontologist, 41*(4): 474-80.

Stuart, M., & Weinrich, M. (2001b). Home is where the help is: Community-based care in Denmark. *J Aging Soc Policy, 12*(4): 81-101.

Wagner, L. (1997). Long-term care in the Danish health care system. *Health Care Management State of the Art Review*, June: 149-156.

doi:10.1300/J031v18n03_03

A Critical Review of Singapore's Policies Aimed at Supporting Families Caring for Older Members

Kalyani K. Mehta, PhD

National University of Singapore

SUMMARY. This article critically examines the family-oriented social policies of the Singapore government aimed at supporting families caring for older members. The sectors focused on are financial security, health, and housing. Singaporeans have been reminded that the family should be the first line of defense for aging families, followed by the community–the state would step in as the last resort. Drawing from recent research and examination of the state policies, the author argues that more should be done to help family caregivers looking after elder relatives. Recommendations for innovative ways to recognize and reward family carers conclude the paper. doi:10.1300/J031v18n03_04 *[Article copies available for a fee from The Haworth Document Delivery Service: 1-800-HAWORTH. E-mail address: <docdelivery@haworthpress.com> Website: <http://www.HaworthPress.com> © 2006 by The Haworth Press, Inc. All rights reserved.]*

KEYWORDS. Family care, Singapore, Asia, policy

[Haworth co-indexing entry note]: "A Critical Review of Singapore's Policies Aimed at Supporting Families Caring for Older Members." Mehta, Kalyani K. Co-published simultaneously in *Journal of Aging & Social Policy* (The Haworth Press, Inc.) Vol. 18, No. 3/4, 2006, pp. 43-57; and: *Family and Aging Policy* (ed: Francis G. Caro) The Haworth Press, Inc., 2006, pp. 43-57. Single or multiple copies of this article are available for a fee from The Haworth Document Delivery Service [1-800-HAWORTH, 9:00 a.m. - 5:00 p.m. (EST). E-mail address: docdelivery@haworthpress.com].

INTRODUCTION

As a city state, Singapore is constrained by its relatively small geographical size, 659.1 square kilometers to be exact, and its lack of natural resources. Singapore's main asset is her people, which totaled four million in June 2000 (Singapore Census of Population, 2000a). The influx of foreign talent, both professional and unskilled, has been encouraged by the government to meet the nation's needs as well as the implications of decreasing birth rates. "Singapore's total fertility rate (TFR) has declined from 1.87 live births per women in 1990 to about 1.50 in 1998. This is partly caused by more young people not marrying or marrying but having fewer or no children" (Ministry of Health, 1999: 32). It is clear, therefore, that the fertility rate has fallen below replacement level–a population needs a TFR of about 2.1 to replace itself. Compounding the effects of falling TFR is the increasing life expectancy of Singaporeans. The life expectancy at birth in 1980 was 70 years for males and 75 years for females. This has increased to 75 years for males and almost 80 years for females in 1999 (Ministry of Health, 1999: 32). The government's effective public health programs largely explain this increase.

The net result is that there will be fewer children to look after aging parents/parents-in-law who will be experiencing longer lives. The aged dependency ratio, calculated on the benchmark of aged as those 65 years and above, has increased from 8.6 per hundred to 10 per hundred over the decade (from 1990 to 2000). On the other hand, the child dependency ratio declined from 33 to 30 per hundred (Singapore Census of Population, 2000b: 5). Demographic statistics on the aging of Singapore's population have been described in detail in other publications (Shantakumar, 1999; Mehta, 2000; Vasoo, Ngiam, & Cheung, 2000); hence, they will not be elaborated in this paper. Singapore's population is aging rapidly, and the impact of this demographic shift will be felt by the health, economic, and welfare sectors most dramatically over the next 30 years.

The phenomenon of an aging demographic profile has been addressed in different innovative ways by developed and developing nations around the world. The "welfare state" model that originated in western countries has certain characteristics that differ from the kinds of welfare-state arrangements prevalent in East Asia. Researchers have discussed the diversity even among nations that espouse the welfare state model, for instance Australia and Canada (see Aspalter, 2002). As compared to the U.K., Singapore follows a minimalist approach to social welfare (Mehta & Briscoe, 2004). Its welfare-oriented policy towards older people in the period 1950 to the 1970s evolved to a developmental-cum-welfare-oriented policy strategy (Mehta, 1997: 33).

SINGAPORE'S SOCIAL POLICY FRAMEWORK

The Singapore government has been consistent in its efforts to create a family-oriented society. One of the key pillars of its national ideology is that "Families are the building blocks of society." The Senior Minister Mr. Goh Chok Tong summarized the national policy on aging population thus: "We want Singaporeans to age with dignity and remain involved in society. We want them to be actively engaged in family and community life. And, in line with the Singapore 21 vision, we must maintain a strong sense of cohesion between the generations. Singapore should be the best home for all generations" (Ministry of Community Development and Sports, 1999: 13).

The Singapore public has been constantly reminded that the family should be the older person's first line of support, followed by the community, that is, voluntary organizations, ethnic-based associations, private foundations, and religious charities. The state would step in to assist these two mechanisms of support when necessary. In other words, the state provides a safety net when seniors are not helped at all by their family members and communities or when the help rendered is inadequate in relation to their needs. The phrase "Many Helping Hands" is captioned by the government to re-iterate that the responsibility for helping the "vulnerable" sectors of the society is shared by many segments of society, underscoring that it is not the responsibility of the state alone to care for them. Mr. Goh Chok Tong described it as a Singaporean approach, which is compassionate yet will not rob the country of its economic competitiveness (*Straits Times*, 1993).

The idea of the family as the first line of defense for the older Singaporean is in tandem with the Asian cultural norms of filial care for one's parents. "In 2000, about 9 in 10 elderly persons above 65 years and over lived with their spouse or children" (Singapore Census of Population, 2000a: 5). This point will be addressed later in this article.

Overall, the Singaporean government's approach has been one of providing subsidized government housing, facilitating and regulating a national provident fund (i.e., Central Provident Fund), and a healthcare delivery system that is a mix of private and public, acute and long-term care, catering to the wealthy as well as the poor.

Older people's developmental needs, for example, social and recreational activities, have been given greater importance with the increase in aging population. The five-year Eldercare Master Plan (FY 2001-2005) of the government allocated a major part of the budget to creating opportunities for volunteer activities for healthy older Singaporeans, gerontological counseling, and caregiver support centers (Ministry of Community Development and Sports, 2001).

This paper makes a critical review of the responses to aging that have been developed to date in this family-oriented framework, and of their capacity to deal with the demographic and social trends set to occur in Singapore over the next 30 years.

OVERVIEW OF SOCIAL POLICIES
TOWARD AGING FAMILIES

While there are many examples of family-oriented policies prevalent in Singapore, such as annual awards for best family-oriented firms/companies, baby bonus schemes to encourage young married couples to start a family, and entry fee concessions for families at tourist attractions, this paper focuses on the family-oriented policies designed to support older people. The focus is on financial security and support, healthcare, housing, and family care. These have been selected because they have direct impacts on older people's and their families' welfare.

Financial Security and Support

The mainstay of financial security of older Singaporeans consists of the Central Provident Fund (CPF) scheme, and where this is inadequate or unavailable for an individual, the family becomes the safety net. The Central Provident Fund, a national social security fund, was established in 1955 to force employees to save a portion of their salaries in a self-managed asset accounts. The employer is also obliged to contribute a certain percentage into the account. At present, employees below age 55 contribute 20% and employers contribute 13% (see the CPF website *www.cpf.gov.sg*). However, the CPF scheme has gradually evolved into "the world's most extensive social policy on assets" (Sherraden et al., 1995: 112).

Each working Singaporean has a CPF account, which is compartmentalized into the ordinary, special, and Medisave accounts. Within certain limits, individuals can expend a portion of their savings on investments, housing, tertiary education for child, and even home protection. The last is a "compulsory mortgage-reducing plan (which) protects members and their families from loss of their homes when members die or are permanently disabled" (Sherraden, 1997: 42). Medisave is a compulsory hospitalization insurance scheme; Medishield is an optional low-cost catastrophic illness insurance that covers individuals till age 80; and the Dependents Protection scheme is an optional term-life insurance scheme that covers members for an insured sum till age 60. All three schemes can be used to cover not only the individual but also his/her family. The premiums are deducted from the individual's monthly contribution to CPF.

The CPF scheme has been criticized for its lack of universal coverage and lack of adequacy of funds for retirement security, especially for the low-income groups (Shantakumar, 1994: 50; Asher 1996: 87; Lee, 1999: 81). The latest National Survey of Senior Citizens (1995) showed that only 33.5% of those over 60 had CPF savings, and of these, 61.6% felt that the CPF savings were inadequate. Historically, many of the current cohorts of elderly did not benefit from the CPF scheme, since it was introduced only in 1955, and Medisave started only in 1984. In the survey, the main reasons cited for inadequate security were the high cost of living, low savings, and high medical costs. Children were the main source of financial support for the majority of the respondents in the survey (Ministry of Health et al., 1995: 22). To be in line with its emphasis on family support, there is an aged-dependent relief provided under the Income Tax assessment. A co-residential child/child-in-law is eligible for S$5000/-tax relief annually, and the non-co-residential counterpart is eligible for S$3500/-annually.

Apart from the CPF, there are two other schemes that act as safety nets for elderly Singaporeans. The first, a Public/Social Assistance scheme, is disbursed by the Ministry of Community Development, Youth and Sports (MCYS) through the Community Development Councils. The elderly formed 86% of the total number of persons who benefited from the scheme in 2003. The rates are not commensurate with the rising rate of inflation in Singapore; for example, an adult can get a maximum monthly allowance of only S$260/- (about US $158/-). A person on public assistance is entitled to free medical services, which are of great help. Secondly, the Medifund scheme is available for poor patients (they must be either Singapore citizens or permanent residents) who are unable to pay their hospital bills. However, the onus for applying for this aid lies on patients, and sometimes they are not aware of Medifund's existence.

The government has opted for a non-welfare state approach from the start, and it is reluctant to make cash payments directly to the needy person. This Singapore-style welfare strategy has been called "supply-side socialism" (*Straits Times, Sunday Review*, 1994) wherein any form of financial assistance is usually provided to the source, for example, to the Housing Development Board for people in rent arrears or to the Nursing Home for subsidy towards frail aged sick. The rationale is to reduce temptation for abuse by the recipient or his/her family members.

Since 1997, the Community Development Councils (CDCs) have started the Interim Financial Assistance Scheme or IFAS. It is a short-term, financial assistance scheme to help a family tide over financial difficulties, for example, in a crisis such as sudden death or retrenchment. In the Asian economic downturn after 1997, many middle-aged workers were laid off and families had to turn to such schemes on a short-term basis till the main bread-winners were re-employed. Skills redevelopment programs were started to help such older workers to get their skills upgraded to fit the new economy. Some of the financial schemes have been streamlined under the Self-Reliance Programme since last year.

In 1996, the Maintenance of Parents' Act was passed by Parliament. The Act is a legal channel open to older Singaporeans who are not being financially supported by their children. The Act is a formal legal mechanism to protect older persons whose adult children may be unfilial and financially neglecting a parent. The Tribunal that reviews the applications (which may be from an older person or even a third party such as the Manager of a Nursing Home) operates under the Ministry of Community Development, Youth and Sports. The relatively low clientele who have approached the Tribunal for Maintenance of Parents (Ministry of Community Development and Sports, 1998) indicates that it functions mainly to serve as a form of preventive strategy against future abandonment by children and to reinforce the social values of filial responsibility.

The Singapore government has sent out a clear signal that family care in old age should be the prevailing norm, a stand that is in keeping with the Asian concept of filial piety. One interesting dimension of this legislation is that an irresponsible parent is not entitled to financial support from adult children. If an elderly parent had abused or deserted his/her children when they were young and in old age he/she tried to file for financial support, the application would be dismissed. However, the adult children have to provide evidence to the Tribunal of the irresponsibility of the parents.

In September 2002, another mechanism under the CPF scheme, Eldershield, was introduced on the opt-out basis to provide financial insurance against disability. It requires a Singaporean between the ages of 40-65 to pay the premiums from his/her Medisave portion of the CPF account, and in the event of having a minimum of three disabilities, he/she is eligible to apply for a subsidy of S$300/- per month for a maximum of five years. The premiums are higher for women than men as a result of their longer life expectancy (see <www.moh.gov.sg> for more details). While the coverage is for life, in fact it is only good for 60 months. The reaction to this scheme has been lukewarm due to the unappealing conditions.

Looking at successive generations of older Singaporeans, future cohorts are likely to have larger amounts that may be withdrawn from their CPF accounts; however, the government has indicated that the Minimum Sum that must be retained will increase over the years. This means that less will be available for spending in retirement, although the Minimum Sum will be available to the individual as a monthly allowance till it is depleted. Since July 2004, S$30,500 has to be retained in the Medisave account for medical expenses in retirement. It is clear that the Medisave amount would not be sufficient to cover all the possible medical expenses in the retirement years, so Singaporeans are urged to purchase private medical insurances.

A serious criticism of the current CPF policy is that there is a lack of financial protection to a surviving widow after her husband dies. According to the rules of the CPF, a member may nominate anyone he/she pleases; the nomination is confidential. Hypothetically, if a woman has never been employed, that is, she has spent her entire life as a homemaker, looking after her husband and children and the elderly parents, she is likely to be financially insecure if her husband has not nominated her as his beneficiary. The reason behind such a policy could be that since it is an individually-managed asset account, the member has a right to choose who he wishes to nominate. Such a policy, however, runs counter to the state's philosophy of the family being the first line of support for the individual.

Health Care

The philosophy adopted by the government is that each person is responsible for maintaining his or her health and well-being, and should save for a rainy day. If this fails, the family should help out. Therefore, the CPF scheme allows children/children-in-law to pay for their parents'/grandparents' hospitalization expenses using their own Medisave savings, but this is not compulsory. However, such usage means that the children may have their own Medisave savings depleted by the time they reach old age.

Currently, according to the Census of Population 2000, singles in the age group 60 years and older form 4% of the population, and the divorced/separated form 2.2%. There are more widowed women than men, while there are more single men than women. In the divorced/separated category, there are more women than men. Poor economic conditions, living alone, and poor health are the common experiences of the singles and the divorced/separated. A newspaper article (*Straits Times*, 2004) titled "No Golden Years for These Women" illustrated the depressive state of many older women who have no family support and no state support. One example cited was that of a single, 70-year-old woman who had attempted suicide twice due to her depressed state; she had to beg for food and money because her financial resources were depleted and mobility problems prevented her from working. These marginalized older people deserve a better deal as they could have spent most of their savings supporting family members, including siblings and ex-husbands, and in their old age they are abandoned by society. The argument being made by some advocacy groups is that the welfare and health policies should be flexible. Such aged Singaporeans who belong to the older immigrant generations should receive a small pension to meet their basic needs, according to these advocates (Shantakumar, 2004).

Healthcare costs form the top concern of older Singaporeans in a recent research conducted by the author (Tan Foundation Project on Needs of Older Singaporeans) as well as focus group discussions conducted by Tsao Foundation. This is not surprising as medical costs are relatively high in Singapore, and a high proportion of elderly do not have any private medical insurance. Their Medisave savings are often low due to their earlier history of low-waged jobs and short span of membership in the CPF scheme. In the first decade (1984-1994), the mandatory contributions were low so the account grew very slowly. Although the government has distributed some of the nation's wealth to these older cohorts through the Medisave top-up scheme, the top-up is uncertain and minimal.

The government allows adult children to buy insurance for their parents using the Medisave fund. Adult children can top up their parents Medisave accounts annually up to S$6,000 without being taxed. A caveat worth mentioning is that adult children have to possess the extra cash to do so, and their willingness is dependent on a positive parent-child relationship. What happens to parents who have strained relationships with their children, or whose children have migrated overseas and have severed all ties as well as filial responsibilities? In the latter case, the Maintenance of Parents Act would not be relevant to their needs because the legal reach would not apply beyond national boundaries. With globalization, the possibility of overseas migration of adult children is a real threat to the well-being of older people in Singapore. Optimistically speaking, the emigrated adult children may send money back, but the physical and emotional care would be lacking. Pessimistically speaking, the older couples would have to fend for themselves financially, emotionally, and physically. Apart from this, the cultural expectations of filial care would be dashed, which psychologically could hasten death (especially if the absent children did not contact the parents at all).

While the system of long term-care has reached a moderate level of development in Singapore (Mehta & Vasoo, 2001), there is a greater demand for affordable nursing homes than there is supply. There is room for a more sophisticated and user-friendly system of community-based and institutional care to meet the needs of the future cohorts of older persons. A study in which the author was the consultant, conducted at the Singapore General Hospital, demonstrated the high levels of stress faced by family caregivers at the point of discharge, largely due to the time taken for arrangements for long-term care. This was partly due to multiple assessments, bureaucratic procedures, and inefficiency. The Integrated Care System (ICS) has helped to some extent to improve effectiveness of transition, but some of the "red tape" could be trimmed.

According to the Census of Population 2000, the impact of immobility is more prevalent among women than among men. Almost 5% of women aged 75 years and older were non-ambulant in 1990 (Singapore Census of Population, 1990), and the figure rose by 2% in 2000. Physical mobility is more of a challenge to older women, and with longer life expectancy, they are likely to have a poorer quality of old age with higher physical dependency. Widowhood combined with physical and financial dependency is a common scenario for the current cohorts of women over 70 years, hence the concern over female elderly suicides in Singapore (Hateley & Tan, 2003). These issues are not dealt with by the current family-oriented policies of the Singapore government, since these policies are not gender-sensitive. Low-income family caregivers also do not get the financial help they need, in lieu of the income tax relief that, ironically, benefits the middle and higher income caregivers.

Housing and Family Care

"The assumption that the care of the young and old is the family's responsibility and traditionally part of the woman's reproductive tasks is also a common feature of families in Southeast Asia. In reality, however, the family system of care has come under tremendous stress and strain as a result of changed work patterns, migration, changes in lifestyles and living arrangements and so forth. And where population control methods have been successful, the burden of care of young and old dependents has become more onerous for smaller families" (Lai & Blake, 1998:186). As mentioned earlier, Singapore has been highly successful in the population-control methods introduced in the middle of the 20th century. The stresses faced by Singaporean families have been documented by many scholars (for example, Quah, 1999). However, in the author's view very few changes have taken place in policies to reduce families' stress until recently. In August 2004, a much awaited key change was the shift to a five-day work week starting with civil servants, a policy change introduced by the incoming Prime Minister Mr. Lee Hsien Loong. Singapore has lagged behind many other developed countries in the legislation of Family Leave for sick parents/parents-in-law, although responsibility for caring of elderly members lies squarely on the shoulders of adult children. Such a policy change would go a long way to reducing the stress of working children/children-in-law. In the United States, such a policy has been in existence for at least a decade (though current U. S. Policy makes provisions only for unpaid leave), as it seems to be a reasonable corollary to child care leave for sick children. (For more information on the Family Medical leave Act in the United States, see "What Role for the Family and Medical Leave Act in Long-Term Care Policy?" in this volume). Many adult children in Singapore find that most of their annual holiday leave is taken up when their elderly relatives fall ill and are hospitalized. Compassionate leave usually covers the employee when a close family member passes away, but the family leave would enable adult children to spend some time with their ill parents. In the context of an aging population, such policies are greatly needed to reduce the stress on adult children, who may be single and therefore may never use any of the paid child care leave! Alternatively, childless married employees would feel that their interests are also being taken care of, since the family leave could replace the sick child care leave from which their colleagues with young children benefit. When stress levels of employees are reduced, productivity is enhanced, and eventually the organization for which they work benefits. Families would simultaneously be strengthened as intergenerational responsibilities could be discharged with less strain and tension.

The high rate of co-residence of older Singaporeans is partly due to the housing policies that provide incentives in various ways. About 90% of Singaporeans live in Housing Development Board (HDB) flats, and this is a statutory board under the government. The Multi-tier housing scheme and Granny flats scheme are examples of priority given to multigenerational family applicants when purchasing their flats. For those who prefer to live near but not under the same roof, the Reside-near Parents scheme offers a grant ranging between S$40,000-50,000 (US$24,000-30,000) for married adult children wishing to purchase a HDB flat near their parents home or parents applying for a flat near (i.e., within two km) of the homes of their married children. A second reason for the high co-residence rate is the high cost of property in Singapore, caused by the tight land constraint.

Government Support for Family Caregivers

While the Singapore government currently provides assistance to self-help groups that support family caregivers, it is small in comparison to the widespread extent of family caregiving and insufficient to address the stress that can arise.

Currently, the National Council of Social Service, a statutory board, provides some financial support for Touch Caregivers Centre (*www.caregivers. org.sg*), which is focused on the needs of caregivers, including caregivers of older kin.

The Ministry of Community Development, Youth and Sports (MCYS) has a Mutual Help Scheme (MHS) that is aimed at facilitating networking among neighboring families with older relatives. This scheme has been in existence for more than a decade; however, publicity is low so not many people are aware of it.

Financial support is also provided by the government towards the Singapore Action Group of Elders (SAGE), a voluntary welfare organization that runs a Counselling Centre specifically targeted at aging families. There is a full-time professional corps of counselors and volunteers trained to manage the telephone hotline for elders and their family members.

The Tribunal of Maintenance of Parents is located at the MCYS. It handles all the applications for the Maintenance of Parents Act. The Family Court handles cases of physical and emotional abuse, which fall under the Women's Charter. According to a recent study, about 100 cases of elder abuse occurred annually for the period 1999-2003 (Sage Counselling Centre, 2004: 27). A non-government organization has been delegated the task of building the necessary protocol to deal with elder abuse cases. Meanwhile, an Elder Protection Team (EPT) has been set up at the MCYS to develop the government strategy in handling this serious social issue. While the numbers are small at the moment, it is speculated that a great deal of under-reporting is likely, and therefore, the appropriate public education and manpower training has to be undertaken.

There is relatively little research done within the Singapore context to study systematically the stress experienced by family members caring for aging relatives. A small-scale study of 61 principal caregivers of homebound elderly patients receiving care from the Hua Mei mobile clinic of Tsao Foundation revealed some salient findings. From the data analysis using Statistical Package for Social Sciences (SPSS), it was shown that a significant inverse relationship existed between level of stress of caregiver and ADL and IADL dependency of care recipient. Caregivers looking after patients suffering from Dementia, Parkinson's disease, and Hypertension were also more likely to be stressed. Finally, female caregivers tended to be more stressed than male caregivers (Mehta & Joshi, 2001). More research is clearly called for in this field to guide policy and attract resources to develop it.

CONCLUSIONS

Bearing in mind the fact that Singapore is aging very rapidly and the physical and psychological stresses of caring for older relatives are high, the level of government support for caregivers needs to be accelerated. As the next five-year Eldercare Masterplan (FY 2006-2010) is under planning, it is strongly recommended that more caregiver support centers be set up, possibly one in each of the five main regions, that is, North, South, East, West, and Central.

The Income Tax relief given for Aged Parents/Grandparents should be complemented by tax rebates for Singaporeans who are co-residing with elderly parents/parents-in-law and earning below a certain level of household income, for example S$2,000. This would be more equitable as they would need the financial help. ·

Regarding the CPF rules on nomination of the beneficiary, it should be made mandatory for the husband (deemed the head of household in a patriarchal society such as Singapore) to get the signature of the wife on the nomination form. To reduce the gender bias, the rule could be applied to both genders.

It is strongly recommended that the government consider a universal pension for all Singaporeans over age 75 in order to distribute the nation's wealth to those who have worked hard to help build the Singapore that exists today. Some criteria could be included, such as that the annual income of the elderly should not be more than two thousand Singapore dollars. This would help to support those elderly without families or if the family members themselves are unemployed/disabled; hence, they may fall outside the scope of current family-focused measures.

Rewards and recognition for the "forgotten army" of family caregivers is grossly overdue in the Singapore context. While the Singapore government may not want to follow the types of policies that exist in Australia such as Carer's allowance or in Europe where it is known as Carer's compensation, there is room for rewards such as medical, transport, or food vouchers. It is well known that the vast majority of family caregivers are women, and giving them free medical tests such as mammograms and bone density scans would be a novel form of reward. Recognition for spousal caregivers is recommended during the Senior Citizens Week in November of each year. Free or subsidized participation at training workshops for caregivers would be an appropriate gift for the winner(s) of such awards. In short, more needs to be done towards a holistic Carer Support Program.

Family-oriented policies need to be made flexible and customized to suit the changing circumstances of the fast transforming Singapore society. Instead of following the "tried and true" path of the past, policymakers should be innovative and daring enough to implement ways to plug the loopholes in the current policies as well as add options for those without families. The momentum must be picked up to create a society that is truly family-oriented in spirit and not just because family-oriented policies presume good economic rationale. The Singapore example can be used by Asian societies that are aging rapidly for policy planning and implementation.

AUTHOR NOTE

Kalyani K. Mehta, PhD, is Associate Professor in the Department of Social Work, National University of Singapore. She can be contacted at the National University of Singapore, Blk AS6 #04-06, 11 Law Link, Singapore 117570 (E-mail: swkkkm@nus.edu.sg).

REFERENCES

Asher, M. (1996). Financing old age in Southeast Asia: An overview. *Southeast Asian Affairs, 23*: 72-98.

Aspalter, C. (2002). *Discovering the Welfare State in East Asia.* Westport, CT: Praeger.

Hateley, L., & Tan, G. (2003). *The Greying of Asia: Causes and Consequences of Aging in Asia.* Singapore: Eastern Universities Press.

Lai, A. E., & Blake, M. (1998). Introduction. *Sojourn: Journal of Social Issues in Southeast Asia, 13*(2): 183-192.

Lee, K. M. (1999). Economic and social implications of aging in Singapore. *Journal of Aging & Social Policy, 10*(4): 73-92.

Mehta, K. (2000). Caring for the elderly in Singapore. In W.T. Liu and H. Kendig (Eds.), *Who Should Care for the Elderly: An East-West Value Divide.* Singapore: Singapore University Press, 249-268.

Mehta, K., & Vasoo, S. (2001). Organization and delivery of long-term care in Singapore: Present issues and future challenges. *Journal of Aging & Social Policy, 13*(2/3): 185-201.

Mehta, K., & Joshi, V. (2001). The long journey: Stress among family carers of older persons in Singapore. *Hong Kong Journal of Gerontology, 15*(1/2): 10-21.

Mehta, K., & Briscoe, C. (2004). National Policy Approaches to Social Care for Elderly in the United Kingdom and Singapore. *Journal of Aging & Social Policy, 16*(1): 485-502.

Mehta, K. (1997). The development of services for the elderly in Singapore: An Asian model. *Asia Pacific Journal of Social Work, 7*(2): 32-45.

Ministry of Community Development (1997). *Annual Report.* Singapore.

Ministry of Community Development and Sports (1998). *Annual Report.* Singapore.

Ministry of Community Development and Sports (1999). *Report of the Interministerial Committee on the Ageing Population.* Singapore.

Ministry of Community Development and Sports (2001). *Eldercare Master Plan* (FY 2001–FY 2005). Singapore.

Ministry of Health, Ministry of Community Development, Ministry of Labour, National Council of Social Service, and Department of Statistics (1995). *National Survey of Senior Citizens.* Singapore.

Ministry of Health (1999). *Report of the Inter-Ministerial Committee on Health Care for the Elderly.* Singapore.

Quah, S. (1999). *Study on the Singapore family.* Singapore: Ministry of Community Development.

Sage Counselling Centre (2004). Say "No" to Elder Abuse. Report by the Golden Life Workgroup on Elder Abuse Prevention. Singapore.

Shantakumar, G. (1994). *The Aged in Singapore.* Census of Population, 1990 Monograph No. 1. Singapore: National Printers.

Shantakumar, G. (1999). Ageing in the City-State Context: Perspectives from Singapore. *Ageing International, 25*(1): 46-58.

Shantakumar, G. (2004). The Position of Older Women: Issues and Policy Challenges in Asian Context. Paper presented at the International Federation on Ageing Conference held in Singapore, September 2004.

Sherraden, M., Nair, S., Vasoo, S., Ngiam, T., & Sherraden, M. (1995). Social policy based on assets: The impact of Singapore's Central Provident Fund. *Asian Journal of Political Science, 3*(2): 112-133.

Sherraden, M. (1997). Provident Funds and Social Protection: The Case of Singapore. In Midgley, J. and Sherraden, M. (Eds.), *Alternatives to Social Security: An International Inquiry.* London: Auburn House, 33-59.

Singapore Census of Population (1990). Advanced Data Release.

Singapore Census of Population (2000a). Advanced Data Release No. 6.

Singapore Census of Population (2000b). A Quick Count.

Straits Times (1993). *Prime Minister spells out welfare policy.* September 12. Singapore.

Straits Times (2004). *No Golden Years for these women.* September 7. Singapore.

Straits Times Sunday Review (1994). *State Welfarism: Singapore Style.* September 18, Singapore.

Vasoo, S., Ngiam, T.L., & Cheung P. (2000). Singapore's ageing population: Social challenges and responses. In D. Phillip's (Ed.) *Ageing in the Asia-Pacific Region: Issues, Policies and Future Trends.* N.Y.: Routledge, 174-193.

www.cpf.gov.sg URL of the Central Provident Fund website, Singapore. Retrieved on December 22, 2004.

www.moh.gov.sg URL of the Ministry of Health website, Singapore. Retrieved on March 25, 2005.

doi:10.1300/J031v18n03_04

Families' Values and Attitudes Regarding Responsibility for the Frail Elderly: Implications for Aging Policy

Nancy Guberman, MSW
University of Quebec

Éric Gagnon, PhD
CSSS de la Vieille Capitale

Jean-Pierre Lavoie, PhD
CSSS Cavendish

Hélène Belleau, PhD
National Institute of Scientific Research

Michel Fournier, MSc
Lise Grenier, BSc
Montreal Public Health Department

Aline Vézina, PhD
Laval University

SUMMARY. This study examines the norms and values associated with care to disabled and frail aging parents, in particular those with regard to the sharing of responsibilities for care between families and formal services, and this within three age cohorts in Quebec, Canada. It is based on a telephone interview of 1,315 people. Factor analysis yielded four factors: (1) family responsibility; (2) uncompromising family obligations; (3) acceptance of services; (4) distrust of services. Analyses of the data indicate that all three age cohorts consider that families have responsibilities for their aging family members, at the same time that they score very high on the acceptance of service scale. This article discusses these seemingly paradoxical results and their implications for aging policy. doi:10.1300/J031v18n03_05 *[Article copies available for a fee from The Haworth Document Delivery Service: 1-800-HAWORTH. E-mail address: <docdelivery@haworthpress.com> Website: <http://www.HaworthPress.com> © 2006 by The Haworth Press, Inc. All rights reserved.]*

[Haworth co-indexing entry note]: "Families' Values and Attitudes Regarding Responsibility for the Frail Elderly: Implications for Aging Policy." Gubermam, Nancy et al. Co-published simultaneously in *Journal of Aging & Social Policy* (The Haworth Press, Inc.) Vol. 18, No. 3/4, 2006, pp. 59-78; and: *Family and Aging Policy* (ed: Francis G. Caro) The Haworth Press, Inc., 2006, pp. 59-78. Single or multiple copies of this article are available for a fee from The Haworth Document Delivery Service [1-800-HAWORTH, 9:00 a.m. - 5:00 p.m. (EST). E-mail address: docdelivery@haworthpress.com].

doi:10.1300/J031v18n03_05

KEYWORDS. Eldercare, family responsibility, formal services, caregiving, values

INTRODUCTION

Research has clearly documented the essential role played by families and friends, mainly women, in the care to community-dwelling disabled elder persons. However, policymakers and researchers alike are voicing fears about the family's capacity to maintain this involvement in care to the elderly in the coming decades (Guberman, 1999; Rosenthal, 2000). These fears are mainly related to demographic trends that point to a growing imbalance between increasing numbers of frail elderly and the reduction of potential caregivers among descendents of the future cohort of elderly, leading to predictions of crisis in terms of who will care for these older people. Weakened marital relations and the multiplication of allegiances as families break up and reconfigure themselves question the capacity of families of the future to support aging parents.

As much of aging policy is predicated on the premise that families are available and desire to provide care for disabled and frail elder members, the possibility that future potential caregivers be less able to assume this work is of serious concern. Indeed, the research on which this article is based is funded through a Quebec government special research program on informal care networks, which states: "The main research preoccupation in terms of informal support concerns, above all, the evolution of the offer of service. Which factors are most likely to intervene and affect the level and proportion of help provided by the informal network?" The government makes numerous references to the various demographic trends mentioned above. Clearly, the Quebec government apprehends a caregiver crunch.

However, this type of analysis does not take into account the norms and values of family solidarity that underlie decisions to care and the ways in which families choose to support aging parents. Two inter-related elements appear to be both changing and significant: the norm of family solidarity and values of autonomy. The gendered nature of family work appears to be in flux as well. Projections and figures are not enough to predict how people will behave. Value systems, family and social norms, and material conditions must all be considered in understanding how family relations are played out.

For some researchers and policymakers, the fact that families and friends continue to provide most of the care to the elderly despite the many documented negative effects to their social and family life, employment, finances, and health is evident proof that feelings of obligation to support family members remain strong. Others, for their part, insist on the erosion of norms of family solidarity in favor of selective and discretionary solidarities based on affective ties and the signification of one's relation to the other (Kellerhals et al., 1994).

Values of autonomy lead to two major forms of family care and assistance to elderly family members (Archbold, 1982; Kellerhals et al., 1994). The first is centered on doing the hands-on care work, the second on having it done by formal services. Some authors consider that these two forms of care reflect two divergent models of autonomy. The first involves family autonomy from formal services and tends to be linked more to a familialist model of family cohesion and functioning characterized by a strong family identity, compulsory and generalized solidarities, rigid forms of interactions, and distrust of the outside world, including reluctance to use services. The second model is based on individual autonomy, of both the elderly parents and other family members. Its focus is on personal autonomy and identity, selective solidarities, negotiated forms of interaction, and use of services outside the family (Clément & Lavoie, 2001; Luna et al., 1996). Formal services allow for a certain balance and help ensure personal autonomy with regard to the family. It appears that older persons increasingly want this autonomy; they do not want to be a burden on family members (Lavoie, 2000; Phillipson, 1997). However, at the same time, they also are very reluctant to be dependent on outside help (Clément et al., 1996).

On the other hand, Attias-Donfut et al. (2002), writing about France, suggest that when faced with a disability, older persons prefer help from their families, while their children (middle-aged adults) and grandchildren (young adults), having grown up in an era of the Welfare State, prefer using public services. However, people with a greater chance of being involved in caregiving tend to favor formal services, as in the case of women.

Indeed, another factor that must be considered in examining how families actualize their responsibilities to aging parents is the gendered nature of care. Women continue to assume most housework and care to family members, although certain studies point to an increased involvement of men (Le Bourdais & Sauriol, 1998).

At another level, several researchers have pointed out that family norms are not specific prescriptions for behavior, but general standards that are reinterpreted, depending on family dynamics and the specific context of the exchange (Finch & Mason, 1993). It is thus important to examine more closely how norms and values of family solidarity are in fact actualized and reinterpreted in the changing contexts of everyday life.

This study's aim is to examine the distribution and the effect of the norms and values associated with care to disabled and frail aging relatives. We particularly examined those norms and values regarding the sharing of responsibilities for care within three age cohorts, in order to inform social policy. Specifically, the study's objectives are to:

1. Determine the distribution of the main norms, values, and attitudes around elder care (family solidarity and responsibility, autonomy, use of formal services) within three age cohorts of Quebecois (70 + years old, 45-59, and 18-30);
2. Identify the care activities that respondents consider family responsibilities;
3. Analyze the impact of contextual variables (relationship among family members, geographical distance, degree of affection, employment, economic status) on the definition of family responsibilities for aging parents.

METHODS

A phone survey was conducted between January and June 2003. (Most of the calls were done between January and March. Because of a software problem, a second wave of calls was needed to survey 150 additional respondents in June 2003.) Respondents answered questions from different scales measuring norms and values. A factorial survey design (Rossi & Anderson, 1982) was used for studying the care activities family should provide and the role of contextual variables on the definition of family responsibilities.

Sample

In all, 1,315 people participated in a 15-minute, on average, telephone interview. The probabilistic sample was taken from randomly generated telephone numbers. Respondents were selected from among private households throughout Quebec with the exception of the territories of Nunavick and the Cree lands around James Bay. Selection criteria included the respondent's ability to understand and speak English or French and being part of one of the three chosen age cohorts, that is

18-30, 45-59, or 70+. When there was more than one eligible respondent in a household, the person was selected based on the age group that had been randomly generated before the call. The response rate was 66.8%.

The final sample was composed of approximately one-third of each of the age cohorts. Specifically, 33% of respondents were aged 18-30 years old, 35.1% were between 45-59 years old, and 31.9% were 70 years and older. Almost a quarter (23.5%) resided on the island of Montreal. The vast majority spoke French (93.2%); the others were English-speaking (6.8%). Sixty percent were women; 46% were married or living in common-law relationships, while 41.8% had post-secondary level schooling (Table 1). Other than a slight under-representation of English-speaking respondents, the sample is comparable to the targeted age groups within the Quebec population.

Survey Instruments

The questionnaire was developed by the researchers and contained three sections. The first part comprised 32 questions, 14 of which were elaborated, based on various scales measuring familism; and 18 were adapted from the *Community Service Attitude Inventory* (CSAI) (Collins et al., 1991), which measures participants' attitudes with regard to formal services. A four-point Likert-type scale going from "complete agreement" to "complete disagreement" was used for answers. The scales were translated to French and retranslated to English to ensure the validity of the translation. The second section presented three vignettes, each followed by seven questions. The goal of the vignettes was to explore the individual's judgment about which types of aid and care should be assumed by a family member in various situations. The last section of the questionnaire included sociodemographic questions. A pre-test was carried out with 100 respondents in January 2003.

Familism. The 15 items measuring familism were adapted from different scales of familism (Bardis, 1959; Cantor & Wilker, 1982; Heller, 1970; Seelbach & Sauer, 1977). Given the age of these scales, the latest dating back to the mid-seventies, and their outdated vision of familism considering the current Quebec context, and given that they were conceived to address the multiple relations of family solidarity, we retained only those items concerning family obligations and those relating to care for and the autonomy of elder family members. The team also developed new items in line with the study objectives.

TABLE 1. Respondents' Sociodemographic Characteristics

Characteristic	n	%
Gender		
Woman	800	60.8
Man	515	39.2
Age group		
18-30	434	33.0
45-59	462	35.1
70+	419	31.9
Language		
French	1226	93.2
English	89	6.8
Civil status		
Single	367	28.0
Married, with partner	604	46.1
Widower	217	16.6
Separated, divorced	122	9.3
Education		
None	4	0.3
Did not complete elementary	89	6.8
Completed elementary	102	7.8
Did not complete high school	220	16.8
Completed high school	346	26.5
College	257	19.7
University	288	22.1

Attitudes with Regard to Service Use. The CSAI is an instrument developed for use with caregivers of community-dwelling elderly suffering from Alzheimer's disease or related dementias. Its aim is to understand and measure caregivers' attitudes with regard to various available services. This scale is comprised of 25 items and 5 sub-scales. For the present study, to reduce the survey length, we retained 17 items by eliminating negative formulations of several questions. Questions were adaptable so they could be answered by non-caregivers and adjusted to the Quebec context with regard to available services.

Types of Care Family Members Should Provide. Three vignettes were presented to each respondent to measure the effect of different contextual variables on attitudes with regard to the type of care family members should provide to an ailing elderly relative. Each vignette described an elderly person in need of care and a relative or friend who could potentially provide this care. The first vignette presented the elderly person and his/her spouse or ex-spouse; the second one, the elderly person and his/her child, step-child, or child-in-law; and the third one, the elderly person and his/her brother or sister, nephew or niece, grandchild, or close friend. Contextual variables referred to the following elements of the scenario: the sex and relationship of the two protagonists, the economic situation of the elder person (low or high income), the geographical distance between the two persons (a few minutes, 30 to 45 minutes, 2 hours travel time), their emotional relationship (close, distant, tense), and whether the relative was employed or not, married and had young children, or not (no child, spouse and child, no spouse and child). All contextual variables were randomly generated, including possible relationships within each category of vignette. Some marginal situations were eliminated: spouses were necessarily of the opposite sex and lived together (the distance variable did not apply); spouses and ex-spouses could not have young children (eliminating the family situation variable). The vignettes contained eight items with 19 possible answers and generated 2,832 possible stories, after elimination of those excluded. After hearing a vignette, respondents had to answer whether or not the targeted person should provide the following types of assistance and care: (1) visit the person and take him/her out; (2) accompany the person to medical and hospital appointments; (3) prepare meals, do housecleaning; (4) give baths, help with dressing; (5) give injections, change wound dressings. Also, if the targeted relative worked, the respondent was asked whether he or she should (6) reduce his/her work time, or (7) move to be closer to the elder person. We employed a fractional replication research plan since not all the vignettes were used.

Analyses

A factor analysis was performed on 31 of the 32 items of the two scales in the questionnaire with M-Plus software (Muthén & Muthén, 2003), using an unweighted least squares estimator (ULS), followed by a VARIMAX rotation. This procedure does not require that answers to items follow an interval scale. Five items were withdrawn because of their low factor loadings. Examination of the scree plot and content considerations led to a decision to retain four factors, which explained 48% of the variance, two from the modified CSAI rather than the original five, and two from our familialism scale. The four factors that were identified are: (1) family responsibility ($\alpha = 0.71$); (2) uncompromising obligations ($\alpha = 0.83$); (3) acceptance of services ($\alpha = 0.62$); (4) distrust of services ($\alpha = 0.80$). The levels of internal consistency are satisfactory given that this is the first validation of these scales and that the judgment with regard to the assistance and care one should offer differs depending on the type of care. Respondents in this study are concerned with eldercare to varying degrees.

The first two factors measure the norms and values underlying family responsibilities and solidarity with regard to frail and ailing community-dwelling elderly family members. The family responsibility factor comprises five items such as "Family members must help their aging relatives in return for what their relatives did for them" and "Older persons should be able to get by without the help of their family." Uncompromising obligations is also comprised of five items and measures the extent to which family responsibility is an obligation no matter what the costs ("Family members should take care of their aging relatives even if it interferes with their work"; "Family members should take care of their aging relatives even if it affects their health."). The two other factors measure attitudes with regard to formal and informal support. Acceptance of formal services measures respondents' inclination to turn to formal services and includes eight items such as "I would feel comfortable using home care services to help me take care of my relative" and "I would not feel comfortable using home care services to help me take care of my relative." Distrust of services comprises nine items such as "My family would think less of me if I were to use home care services" and "I would be afraid of having home care personnel take care of my relative," which measure non-confidence in formal services, perceived social image for using services, and preference for support from family and friends. For each subscale, we calculated average item scores based on a four-point Likert-type scale where 4 indicates that the construct is accentuated.

Linear regressions were performed on the four subscales to compare our three cohorts while controlling for variables that could potentially influence values and attitudes toward family responsibilities and formal services. The controlled confounding variables are gender, education, marital status, needing care, and involvement in caregiving.

In the case of the vignettes, logistical regression analyses were performed to evaluate the impact of the contextual variables on the types of care one should offer a frail elderly relative or friend.

Types of assistance and care are the dependent variables (dichotomized: yes or no). The eight context variables are the main independent variables. Because we once again wanted to compare the three cohorts, we used the same independent variables as in the linear regressions.

RESULTS

Family Responsibility Values and Attitudes to Service Use

Analyses of the data indicate that all three age cohorts consider that families have responsibilities for their aging family members. Indeed, 84.1% of all respondents indicated total or general agreement with the statement, "Family members must help their aging relatives in return for what their relatives did for them," and 81% with, "It is the duty of family members to take care of their aging relatives." With regard to the statement, "people are just as responsible for their elder parents as they are for their own children," 70% of respondents indicated agreement. However, percentages dropped to 42.7% in answer to a statement regarding co-residency with an ailing elder relative ("When an older person is unable to live at home without assistance, it is better that they live with one of their children"). The average mean scores for the items pertaining to family responsibility are high, indicating that respondents generally agree with the idea that families are responsible for the well-being of elderly members (Table 2). It should be noted, however, that this agreement decreases with age. The youngest cohort is more in agreement with this idea (average score = 3.1) than 45-59 year olds (average score = 2.8) and than those 70 and older (average score = 2.5) who are the most lukewarm with regard to norms of family responsibility.

However, when questioned more specifically with regard to the notion of responsibility, respondents began to put limits on the level of concessions family members should have to make to assure care. Respondents were divided regarding whether "Family members should care even if it interferes with their social life," with 57.6% showing complete or general support for this idea. This is not the case for other consequences of care. Only 38.9% support the idea that family members should provide care even if it leads to family conflicts, while proportions fall to 27.9% when it hurts their professional lives and 12.0% if it is harmful to their health or it is done to the detriment of their children. . Once again, globally, the younger cohort is more familist, showing more openness to assuming certain inconveniences linked to elder care (disturbing one's social life, affecting one's health, etc.). For this scale, the average score for 18-30 year olds is 2.2 compared to 1.9 for those 70+ (Table 2).

In contrast to the questions from the family responsibility and obligations scales, questions from the acceptance and distrust of services

TABLE 2. Average Scores and Standard Deviation of Subscales by Age Cohort

SUBSCALE	SCORES [1]					
	18-30 years		45-59 years		70 years +	
	$\overline{X}$	s	$\overline{X}$	s	$\overline{X}$	s
Family responsibility	3.1	.49	2.8	.64	2.5	.68
Uncompromising obligations	2.2	.61	2.1	.71	1.9	.77
Acceptance of services	3.3	.40	3.4	.39	3.5	.42
Distrust of services	1.9	.54	1.7	.52	1.9	.63

[1] Scores vary from 1 to 4: (1) completely disagree; (2) somewhat disagree; (3) somewhat agree and (4) completely agree.

scales measure respondents' attitudes rather than their general opinions regarding family responsibility for care.

Answers to the acceptance of services scale show that despite high levels of agreement with regard to norms of family responsibility, the vast majority of respondents (95.5%) "Would feel comfortable using home care services to help take care of [their] relative," and 95.2% would "willingly use services offered by the government." Indeed, 86.8% feel that "when an older person is unable to live at home without assistance, it is better that they live in a seniors residence or nursing home," as compared to 42.7% who approved the idea that they should move in with a child. Results indicate that most respondents in all age cohorts would not be, and in the case of current caregivers are not, reticent to turn to services. Acceptance of services seems to increase with age, with average scores rising from 3.3 in the youngest cohort to 3.5 in the oldest (Table 2).

In line with this openness, only one respondent out of four (24.4%) believes that family members should take on all the care for their aging relatives without asking for help outside the family. Few feel that they should avoid using services (22.5%); that they would be anxious for their relative's safety if left with a service provider (24.9%); that they would have difficulty trusting services (18.8%); or that their family would think less of them for using services (11.4%). However, acceptance of help from formal services does not seem to extend to friends: 86.9% of respondents prefer turning to home care services rather than asking friends for help. Also, only 39% would prefer to seek help from their family rather than use home care services. Average scores for distrust of services appear quite low, especially among the 45-59 years old cohort (average score of 1.7 versus 1.9 for the two other cohorts–Table 3).

All differences among cohorts remain significant even when controlled for gender, education, civil status, needing help, and experience in caregiving (data not shown in this paper).

Vignettes: Types of Care and Context Variables

With the vignettes, respondents were asked to specify the types of care that a targeted family member or friend should offer (Table 3). Taking the sample as a whole, approximately two thirds of respondents think that the targeted family member should visit the disabled person or take him or her out, or should accompany the disabled person to medical or hospital appointments. Family responsibility is clearly less important regarding instrumental tasks and personal or nursing care, with only 20% to 30% in agreement that the targeted member should help with meals and housecleaning, bathing and dressing, giving injections, or changing wound dressings. Around one in seven respondents would have the targeted member move closer to the disabled person or consider reducing work time to care.

When we examine how modifying different aspects of context had impact on respondents' answers, we find that the gender and the income level of the disabled elderly person have no effect on respondents' answers (Table 4). However, the relationship between the two protagonists, the family and professional situation of the targeted member, the quality of the emotional relation, and geographical proximity are all elements that reinforce or limit agreement with their involvement in the

TABLE 3. Care Activities Targeted Family Member Should Provide by Age Cohort

CARE ACTIVITIES	18-30 years		45-59 years		70 years +		Total
	%[1]	OR[2]	%	OR	%	OR	%
Visits and outings	73.5	1.6*	63.0	.86	65.6	-	67.3
Medical, hospital appointments	64.8	.72*	58.9	.53*	69.2	-	64.1
Meals, house cleaning	28.9	.77	29.3	.70*	36.3	-	31.3
Bathing, dressing	24.6	.92	20.6	.65*	28.4	-	24.3
Injections and change dressings	22.9	1.2	16.9	.81	22.1	-	20.6
Move closer	17.4	.78	10.7	.46*	21.8	-	16.4
Reducing work time	13.4	.62	12.8	.59	17.9	-	14.5

[1]% of positive answers, i.e., targeted family member should provide the care activity
[2]Odds Ratio when controlling for gender, education, civil status, care need, caregiving experience and context variables (see Table 4). 70 years and + is the reference category.
* p < 0.01

different care activities. Spouses, compared to ex-spouses, for example, are expected to a greater extent to assume most care activities and to reduce work time (Odds Ratio (OR) of 7.1 for men and 3.9 for women). Those who live nearby, compared to those who live more than two hours away (OR of 1.5 to 1.9), are expected to visit and are more frequently expected to help with household chores. There is a smaller expectation that those who have children move if they live far away (OR of .48 to .53 to childless family member) and that those who have close emotional relationships be more present than those with tense relationships.

Regarding differences among the three cohorts, the portrait is different from that based on the scales. People in the 70+ group have higher expectations of the targeted family member than those in the 45-59 year old group for many of the support activities: medical and hospital appointments, meals and house cleaning, bathing and dressing (Table 3). They also consider more often than the middle group that a targeted family member living far away should move closer to his/her disabled older relative. For most activities, although the odds ratios are generally not significant, the youngest cohort falls between the two others. However, younger respondents indicate more frequently that the targeted person should visit or take the older person out (OR = 1.6) but are less likely than the 70 + group to suggest that the targeted member accompany the older person to medical appointments (OR = .72).

DISCUSSION

How can we understand the somewhat paradoxical results whereby respondents indicate strong family values, with 80% agreeing with the statement that it is the duty of family members to care for elderly parents, while at the same time they also strongly embrace the idea of using formal services? To some extent, this can be explained by attempting to understand what the value of family responsibility means for our respondents. Based on their answers to the vignettes, where respondents were asked to indicate which types of care should be offered by a specific family member or friend to a frail elderly person, it would appear that family responsibility extends to the offering of emotional and moral support and accompanying the older person to appointments. On the other hand, the vast majority of respondents show much openness to delegating instrumental, physical, and nursing tasks to home care services or long-term care homes. It should be noted that some studies—

TABLE 4. Logistic Regression on Care Activity–Odds Ratios for Context Variables

Context variables		Visits and outings	Medical, hospital appointments	Meals, house cleaning	Bathing, dressing	Injections and change dressings	Move	Reducing work time
				Care activity				
Gender (care recipient)	Woman	.97	.96	.96	.90	.97	1.2	.91
	Man	–	–	–	–	–	–	–
Relationship	Husband	NA	12.7*	13.2*	9.9*	3.5*	NA	7.1*
	Wife	NA	7.5*	16.4*	8.9*	3.4*	NA	3.9*
	Ex-husband	1.3	1.3	.97	1.1	.81	.93	.98
	Ex-wife	–	–	–	–	–	–	–
	Son	4.6*	2.1*	1.7	1.4	1.4	1.8	.76
	Daughter	3.8*	1.7	1.3	1.2	1.6	1.9	.85
	Step-son	2.3*	1.3	.95	.67	.99	1.9	1.2
	Step-daughter	1.3	1.0	.96	.67	.87	1.0	.70
	Son-in-law	1.5	.97	.80	.38*	.64	1.8	.45
	Daughter-in-law	1.8*	1.4	1.3	.82	.84	.79	.91
	Brother	2.0*	1.5	.89	.74	.93	1.6	.69
	Sister	1.6	1.2	1.9*	1.4	1.2	1.7	.65
	Grandson	2.5*	1.0	.83	.51	.68	.71	.57
	Granddaughter	2.0*	1.1	.97	.79	.66	1.4	.44
	Nephew	1.5	.91	.73	.89	1.2	1.5	.74
	Niece	1.2	.71	1.1	.99	1.2	.72	.46
	Close male friend	4.7*	1.6	1.2	.96	.81	1.6	.61
	Close female friend	5.5*	1.5	1.5	.96	1.1	1.6	.64
Quality of relationship	Close	4.6*	2.4*	1.5*	1.6*	1.4*	1.3	1.1
	Distant	1.4*	1.2	1.1	1.0	.95	1.1	.92
	Tense	–	–	–	–	–	–	–
Family situation (caregiver)	Single parent	.85	.58*	.63*	.69*	.62*	.53*	.82
	Married with children	.86	.57*	.67*	.68*	.61*	.48*	.99
	No dependent child	–	–	–	–	–	–	–
Geographical distance	A few minutes	1.9*	2.9*	2.7*	2.0*	1.7*	NAP	.73
	30 to 45 minutes	1.5*	2.2*	1.5*	1.3	1.3	.69*	.81
	2 hours	–	–	–	–	–	–	–
Work	Full time	.85	.57*	.59*	.78*	.81	.82	NA
	No employment	–	–	–	–	–	–	NA
Income (care recipient)	Well off	1.0	.91	.93	1.0	1.0	.94	.89
	Low income	–	–	–	–	–	–	–

* p < 0.01

such as Lavoie, 2000–indicate that escorting an older person for medical visits comprises more than the act of transporting them. It is also a way for family members to monitor the situation, obtain medical information, and offer emotional support.

Put succinctly, for our respondents, family responsibility means, "being there" for the older family member, that is, ensuring his or her emotional well-being, sociability, and continued integration in society through contacts with the outside world. Family responsibility can also mean monitoring the person's health and safety. Families are particularly well-suited to assuming these aspects of care as they are best situated to ensure the singularity of their members, because the person is "my mother" or "my brother" and not just a home care client or another case of dementia. Because of their common history and emotional bonds, family members can be expected to demonstrate their affection for the older person, protect his or her dignity, and pay respect in reciprocity for what the older person has done for them. Given this, one can better understand why answers in the vignettes define family responsibility less in terms of instrumental activities and more in terms of a social and emotional presence

But even with this more circumscribed understanding of family responsibility, this responsibility has its limits, given the low scores on obligations. Even if family responsibility is understood as mainly affective and emotional, it should not cause undue hardship on family members or interfere too much with their own lives. Family and friends, for example, should not have to move or reduce employment to care for a frail elderly person, nor should care responsibilities impact negatively on their health or interfere with their relations with their own children.

Another or complementary interpretation of these findings is elucidated by the intergenerational ambivalence approach (Luescher & Pillemer, 1998), which advances that parents and children experience ambivalence in the face of growing support needs by the former because of opposing pressures for freedom from the parent-child relationship (Cohler & Allergott, 1995). And, we would add, because of the influence of the autonomist model with its focus on the individual's quest for autonomy and resistance to normative relationships and duties to others (Clément & Lavoie, 2000; Luna et al., 1996). Thus, respondents are conceivably torn between the contradictory normative expectations of autonomy and family solidarity leading them to score high on both the scale of family responsibility and the acceptance of services scale as they juggle norms of obligation and reciprocity and those of self-actualization.

In examining the responses to the vignettes, it appears that expectations with regard to family solidarity are not identical for all concerned but are modulated by the context of the frail elderly person and that of the potential caregiver and this for the entire range of activities. For example, there appears to be a separate logic at work in the case of spouses. Indeed, the normative expectations around conjugal solidarity and mutual support appear to be very high and over-ride other exhortations regarding individual realization and autonomy. Spouses of both sexes are seen as having specific responsibilities to each other in old age, with approximately three quarters of respondents indicating they should make meals or do housework for a disabled partner, and just over 60% that they should help with bathing and dressing or undressing. It is also expected by 50% of respondents that a husband should reduce work time to care for his wife, while only 39% expect the same from the wife.

Other elements of context such as living near-by, being childless, or having a positive affective relationship with the frail elderly relative lead to higher expectations with regard to involvement in care, in particular, moving nearer to the elderly person. One might postulate that geographical and affective proximity are sex-related conditions with women tending to be both physically and emotionally closer to parents. To that extent, although the sex of the targeted family member in the vignettes was never significant, expectations are the same for men and women, and even somewhat higher for men with regard to traveling (visits and appointments); gendered expectations may be hidden behind the belief that those living closer and with closer affective relationships should provide more care.

As presented in Table 2, young people (18-30) feel significantly more strongly about family responsibility, are more uncompromising with regard to the family's role, less likely to accept services, and are more distrustful of services than the older cohorts. This finding corresponds to similar results from the U.K. and Israel (where the youngest group included people between the ages of 25 and 49) but differ from Spain and Germany, where this group had fewer familistic values than the older groups (Lowenstein & Daatland, 2004). The former two countries have welfare regimes and familial cultures that more resemble Quebec's regimes and cultures than those of the latter two.

A finding of stronger values of family responsibility among the youngest age cohort might lead to optimism with regard to the future of caregiving, notably to the baby-boomer generation, for whom the younger cohort comprises a bank of potential caregivers. However, two elements lead us to a more cautious interpretation of the findings. Firstly, values in younger cohorts have been shown to be slightly more unstable than those of older cohorts, becoming more similar to those of the older cohorts as the younger group ages (Roberts & Bengston, 1999). Secondly, in our own study, the differences in the younger cohort's values compared with those of the other age cohorts are less strong in the analysis of responses to the vignettes. It would appear that when asked general questions about family responsibility younger respondents have a more "idealized" vision of family solidarity and tend to hold high expectations of family members. However, when confronted with the concrete nature of this solidarity, ADLs, IADLs, and nursing care, as outlined in the vignettes, younger respondents tend to put more limits on family responsibility and become less uncompromising about family obligations. Another area where expectations of change are not supported by our findings concerns turning to friends for care. Friends are sometimes seen as a potential group that could replace family members in caregiving for future cohorts of frail elderly. However, the vast majority of our respondents of all age cohorts seems very reluctant to call on friends.

CONCLUSION

Our study offers little empirical evidence that the first choice of most frail elderly is to depend on family for hands-on caregiving, nor that most family members would freely and willingly choose to do so. On the contrary, it points to increased openness to delegating responsibilities to formal services. It would seem that values of individual autonomy and independence from others structure current family solidarities in Quebec. Respondents indicate that they are willing to provide support to frail elderly family members or friends but that this support is circumscribed, has its limits, and takes place within particular family contexts. This is in marked opposition to the foundation of most aging and home care policy. As Kane and Penrod (1995) indicate, there is a range of policy options with regard to family care open to governments. These run the gamut from "benign neglect," where no policy is a de facto policy with underlying values of private responsibility for care, to a policy of high levels of available and accessible formal care to relieve families of much of the hands-on responsibility of care. In between there are policies aimed more at shoring up caregivers to ensure that they are able to maintain their roles and pursue high levels of care, than at replacing them or sharing the responsibility. This latter approach, which some have called the "caregiver as resource" (Guberman & Maheu, 2002) or the "caregiver as co-worker" approach (Twigg, 1988), gives rise to policies and practices aimed at increasing the caregiver's ability and competency to support his or her relative, while recognizing the importance of ensuring their emotional and psychological well-being. However, this preoccupation for the caregiver's well-being is, in the end, just a means of ensuring his or her on-going participation in care. An analysis of Quebec home care policy reveals that family care is its lynch pin. Residential care is available only to the extent that the family defaults on its responsibility and is not offered as an acceptable alternative to home care. Support to caregivers is offered as a way of preventing institutionalization (Lavoie et al., 2003). To that extent, home care services are quite minimal–Quebec spends the lowest per capita amount for these services of all the Canadian provinces–despite the fact that in the most recent home care policy adopted in 2003, caregivers are presented as partners and potential clients of the system who have the right to take on care on the basis of an informed decision, whose involvement is voluntary, and can be questioned at any time. In stark contrast, the under funding of the system obliges families to do much more than they often want to do or to take on care activities they feel should be the responsibility of the public sector (Gagnon et al., 2002). (In Quebec, front-line health and social services, including home care, were taken over by the state and became public services in the early 1970s. As such they have been offered universally and free, although availability and accessibility have been a problem. There is now a move to remove homemaker services [ADLs and IADLs] from the basket of free services.)

The contradictions between policy orientations and the values of the population, as revealed in this study, can play themselves out in several ways. The state may be able to continue imposing its orientation and ensuring that eldercare is mainly assumed by family and friends who have few options but to fill the gap left by inadequate state intervention. In this scenario, the state will continue to claim concern about caregiver burn-out and provide a limited number of services aimed at supporting caregivers, such as occasional respite, support groups, and some individual counseling, without substantially modifying the division of responsibility for elder care.

However, given the values held by respondents in this study, it is more likely that current and future caregivers, particularly non-spouses, will look for substitutes to their own hands-on caregiving and to the extent that they have the financial means to do so, turn to the for-profit private and community sectors. In Quebec, this would mean a setback in terms of the universality of free and adequate health and social services and lead to greater inequalities among families. Quite likely, as more families assume out-of-pocket expenses for care, they will be increasingly reluctant to pay high income taxes for public services, thus further broadening the gap between families with and without means to pay for care.

A third scenario would see caregiver advocacy groups, women's groups, and seniors' and disabled persons' rights groups rally public opinion so that the discourse of current home care policy be made a reality and that caregiving be the result of selected solidarities and a negotiated division of responsibilities between families and the state.

AUTHOR NOTES

Nancy Guberman, MSW, is Professor in the School of Social Work at the University of Quebec. She is also scientific director of the Gerontology Research Centre at the CSSS Cavendish. As corresponding author, Dr. Guberman can be contacted at the School of Social Work, University of Quebec, Montreal, P.O. Box 8888, Station Centreville, Montreal, Quebec, H3C 3P8 (E-mail: guberman.nancy@uqam.ca).

Jean-Pierre Lavoie, PhD, is a senior researcher at the Gerontology Research Centre at the CSSS Cavendish.

Michel Fournier, MSc, is a researcher, and Lise Grenier, BSc, is a research assistant, both with the Montreal Public Health Department.

Éric Gagnon, PhD, is a senior researcher at the CSSS de la Vieille Capitale.

Aline Vézina, PhD, is Professor of Social Work at Laval University.

Hélène Belleau, PhD, is at the National Institute of Scientific Research and Scientific Director of the Research Center at the CSSS Nord de I'Ile/St-Laurent.

The research on which this paper is based was funded by a special program on aging of the FQRSC (Fonds québécois de recherché sur la société et la culture–Quebec Fund for Research on Society and Culture).

REFERENCES

Archbold, P. G. (1982). An analysis of parentcaring by women. *Home Health Care Services Quarterly, 3*(2): 5-25.

Attias-Donfut, C., Lapierre, N., & Segalen, M. (2002). *Le nouvel esprit de famille.* Paris: Éditions Odile Jacob.

Bardis, P. (1959). A familism scale. *Journal of Marriage and the Family, 21*: 340-341.

Cantor, M., & Wilker, L. (1982). Parent-child relations. In D. Mangen, & W. Peterson (Eds.), *Research instruments in social gerontology, Vol.2: Social roles and social participation* (pp. 115-185). Minneapolis: University of Minnesota Press.

Clément, S., Grand, A., & Grand-Filaire, A. (1996). Aide aux personnes vieillissantes. In J. C. Henrard, S. Clément, & F. Derriennic (Éds.), *Vieillissement, santé, société* (pp. 163-189). Paris: Les éditions INSERM.

Clément, S., & Lavoie, J. P. (2001). L'interface formel-informel au confluent de rationalités divergentes. In J. C. Henrard, O. Firbank, S. Clément, M. Frossard, J. P. Lavoie, & A. Vézina (Eds.), *Personnes âgées dépendantes en France et au Québec. Qualité de vie, pratiques et politiques* (pp. 97-119). Paris: INSERM.

Cohler, B., & Altergott, K. (1995). The family of the second half of life. Connecting theories and findings. In R. Blieszner, & V. Hilkevitch (Eds.), *Handbook of Aging and the Family*. Westport: Greenwood Press.

Collins, C., Stommel, M., King, S., & Given, C. W. (1991). Assessment of the attitudes of family caregivers toward community services. *The Gerontologist, 31*: 756-761.

Finch, J., & Mason, J. (1993). *Negotiating Family Responsibilities*. London & New York: Tavistock/Routledge.

Gagnon, E., Guberman, N., Côté, D., Gilbert, C., Thivièrge, N, & Tremblay, M. (2002). Les soins à domicile dans le contexte du virage ambulatoire. *L'Infirmière du Québec, 10*: 12-24.

Garant, L., & Bolduc, M. (1990). *L'aide par les proches: mythes et réalité*. Québec: Ministère de la Santé et des Services sociaux, Direction de la planification et de l'évaluation.

Giddens, A. (1991). *Modernity and self-identity*. Stanford: Stanford University Press.

Guberman, N. (1999). *Caregivers and Caregiving: New Trends and their Implications for Policy*, Report prepared for Health Canada, mimeo, 127p.

Guberman, N., & Maheu, P. (2002). Conceptions of family caregivers: Implications for professional practice. *Canadian Journal of Aging, 21*: 25-35.

Heller, P. L. (1970). Familism scale: A measure of family solidarity. *Journal of Marriage and the Family, 32*: 73-80.

Kane, R. A., & Penrod, J. D. (1995). In Search of Family Caregiving Policy: General Considerations. In R. Kane & J. D. Penrod (Eds), *Family Caregiving in an Aging Society*. Thousand Oaks, CA: Sage.

Kellerhals, J., Coenen-Huther, J., von Allmen, M., & Hagmann, H. (1994). Proximité affective et entraide entre générations: la "génération-pivot" et ses pères et mères. *Gérontologie et Société, 68*: 98-112.

Lavoie, J. P. (2000). *Familles et soutien aux parents âgés dépendants*. Paris: L'Harmattan.

Lavoie, J-P, Grand, A., Guberman, N., & Andrieu, S. (2003). Les dispositifs d'action sur l'aide de l'entourage en France et au Québec. *Gérontologie et Société, 107*: 109-129.

Le Bourdais, C. & Sauriol, A. (1998). *La part des pères dans la division du travail domestique au sein des familles canadiennes*. Montreal: INRS-Urbanisation, Études et documents.

Lowenstein, A., & Daatland, S. O. (2004). Filial Norms and Family Support to the Old-Old (75+) in a Comparative Cross-National Perspective (The OASIS Study). Paper presented at 57th Annual Scientific Meeting of the Gerontological Society of America, Washington, November.

Luescher, K., & Pillemer, K. (1998). Intergenerational ambivalence: A new approach to the study of parent-child relations in later life. *Journal of Marriage and the Family, 60*: 413-425.

Luna, I., de Ardon, E. T., Mi Lin, Y., Cromwell, S. L., Phillips, L. R., & Russell, C. K. (1996). The Relevance of Familism in Cross-Cultural Studies of Family Caregiving. *Western Journal of Nursing Research, 18*: 267-283.

Muthén, L. K., & Muthén, B. O. (2003). *Mplus user's guide (second edition)*. Los Angeles, CA: Muthén & Muthén.

Phillipson, C. (1997). La prise en charge des parents âgés en Grande-Bretagne: Perspectives sociologiques. *Lien social et Politiques-RIAC, 38*: 165-173.

Roberts, R. E. L., & Bengston, V. L. (1999). The Social Psychology of Values: Effects of Individual Development, Social Change, and Family Transmission over the Life Span. In C. D. Ryff and V. W. Marshall (Eds.), *The Shelf and Society in Aging Processes* (pp. 453-482). New York: Springer Publishing Co.

Rosenthal, C. (2000). Aging families: Have current changes and challenges been "oversold"? In E. M. Gee, & G. M. Gutman (Eds.), *The Overselling of Population Aging. Apocalyptic Demography, Intergenerational Challenges, and Social Policy* (pp. 43-65). Oxford: Oxford University Press.

Rossi, P. H., & Anderson, A. B. (1982). The Factorial Survey Approach: An Introduction. In P. H. Rossi, & S. L. Nock (Eds.), *Measuring Social Judgments: The Factorial Survey Approach* (pp.15-67). Beverly Hills: Sage Publications.

Seelbach, W. C., & Sauer, W. J. (1977). Filial responsibility expectations and morale among aged parents. *The Gerontologist, 17*: 492-499.

Twigg, J. (1988). Models of carers: How do social care agencies conceptualize their relationship with informal carers. *International Social Policy, 18*: 53-66.

doi:10.1300/J031v18n03_05

THE UNITED STATES

Commentary:
What Role for the Family and Medical
Leave Act in Long-Term Care Policy?

Steven K. Wisensale, PhD

University of Connecticut

SUMMARY. The Family and Medical Leave Act provides unpaid leave but a key component is its intergenerational structure, permitting employees to take time off from work to care for an infant as well as an ill elderly parent. However, in an effort to provide paid leave, 23 of 28 states dropped the elder care provision in new initiatives introduced between 2000 and 2003. This article argues that in reforming leave policy in the future, the leave should be paid, remain intergenerational, cover more workers, and be adaptable to changing family patterns in an aging society. Also discussed is California's paid leave law, which meets these criteria. doi:10.1300/J031v18n03_06 *[Article copies available for a fee from The Haworth Document Delivery Service: 1-800-HAWORTH. E-mail address: <docdelivery@haworthpress.com> Website: <http://www.HaworthPress.com> © 2006 by The Haworth Press, Inc. All rights reserved.]*

[Haworth co-indexing entry note]: "Commentary: What Role for the Family and Medical Leave Act in Long-Term Care Policy?" Wisensale, Steven K. Co-published simultaneously in *Journal of Aging & Social Policy* (The Haworth Press, Inc.) Vol. 18, No. 3/4, 2006, pp. 79-93; and: *Family and Aging Policy* (ed: Francis G. Caro) The Haworth Press, Inc., 2006, pp. 79-93. Single or multiple copies of this article are available for a fee from The Haworth Document Delivery Service [1-800-HAWORTH, 9:00 a.m. - 5:00 p.m. (EST). E-mail address: docdelivery@haworthpress. com].

KEYWORDS. Caregivers, family leave, intergenerational policies, long-term care

INTRODUCTION

The Family and Medical Leave Act (FMLA) of 1993 was the first bill signed by newly elected President Bill Clinton. Its adoption marked the end of eight years of congressional debate and two vetoes by his predecessor, George Bush. It allows a worker to take up to 12 weeks of unpaid leave in any 12-month period for the birth or adoption of a child, to care for a sick child, spouse, or parent with a serious health condition, or for the worker's own health condition. The law further guarantees job security in that an employee is entitled to return to the same or comparable job and requires the employer to maintain health benefits as if the employee never took leave. The law applies only to companies with 50 or more employees and to workers who have been employed for at least one year or 1,250 hours. It also allows a company to deny leave to a salaried employee who falls within the highest 10% of the company's payroll if the worker's leave would create "substantial and grievous injury" to the business operations. It requires employees to notify their employers prior to taking leave and permits the employer to request medical opinions to justify the employee's absence. And, in the event a worker elects not to return to work after the leave expires, the employer may require the employee to repay all health care premiums that were paid during his or her absence.

By the time Bill Clinton signed the FMLA into law in 1993, 34 states had already adopted some form of leave policy, with several producing comparable or stronger legislation than the federal version (Wisensale, 2001). Twenty-three states covered both private and state employees; eleven states applied their policies to state employees only. Nineteen states gave time off for pregnancy and childbirth, while fifteen states had adopted broader types of legislation, permitting leave for more general family matters. There was also much variation among the states in duration of leave and the size of companies to which the law applied.

With respect to structure, the FMLA has three major characteristics that place it in sharp contrast to typical models in other industrialized nations. One, it is unpaid. All industrialized countries, except Australia and the United States, provide some form of wage replacement for those taking leave. Two, the American model has a *family* focus. That is, unlike its European counterparts that are designed for new *parents*, the

U.S. law is *intergenerational* in structure, thus allowing time off from work for the birth or care of a child as well as care for an elderly parent. And three, unlike other industrialized countries, the United States links eligibility for leave to company size (50 + employees). Consequently, the FMLA applies only to about 6% of the corporations and 60% of the labor force.

Because the FMLA is often discussed in terms of child care, little attention has been devoted to its potential for addressing major long-term care demands. However, as the baby boom generation retires and is afflicted with multiple chronic illnesses 15 to 20 years later, more families will be called upon to address the personal health care needs of their elderly relatives. Between 2000 and 2002, more than 20 states introduced legislation to provide paid leave to family caregivers through the use of state unemployment insurance trust funds. However, almost all of the state initiatives limited the coverage to "baby care." In short, the original intergenerational structure of the law is slowly being dismantled by well-intentioned state legislators who are seeking to provide paid leave. This can be particularly problematic in light of future projections of the long-term care needs of an aging population.

That said, this paper addresses four research questions. First, who is using the FMLA and why? But more specifically, to what extent has the FMLA been used by family caregivers to provide assistance to the elderly? Second, if our past is our future, what do we know about the history of family caregiving and what role will adult children play in the future in addressing the needs of their elderly parents? Third, what are the costs of supporting or not supporting family care of the elderly and how should the FMLA be factored into such cost assessments? And fourth, what are the major shortcomings in the existing FMLA with respect to care of the elderly, and how should states address these weaknesses as they put forth initiatives to provide paid leave?

WHO IS USING THE FMLA AND WHY?

Since the FMLA was implemented on August 5, 1993, the Department of Labor has evaluated it twice–in 1995 and 2000. On April 30, 1996, the Commission on Leave issued its first report: *A Workable Balance: Report to Congress on Family and Medical Leave Policies*. The 314-page document concluded that the FMLA had a positive impact on employees overall and was not the burden on businesses that some had predicted. Ninety percent of companies covered by the law reported no negative impact. "For most employers, compliance is easy, the costs are non-existent or small and the effects are minimal," states the report. "Most periods of leave are short, most employees return to work, and reduced turnover seems to be a tangible effect" (Commission on Leave, 1996).

In more specific terms, between 1993 and 1995 nearly 15 million people used the Family and Medical Leave Act for either personal reasons or to care for a family member. Table 1 shows the percentage of all leave-takers and their reasons for taking leave in descending order as reported in the Department of Labor's 1995 and 2000 surveys.

It was also reported that 3.4% of employees who needed leave did not take it. Of those, about 66% indicated that the reason they did not use the FMLA was that they could not afford it (Commission on Leave, 1996). Unknown is the number of those who were caring for the elderly but could not afford to take leave.

The second major evaluation of the FMLA completed by the Department of Labor was published in 2000. In *Balancing the Needs of Families and Employers: Family and Medical Leave Surveys*, the Department of Labor reported that the total number of workers who took leave under the FMLA increased from 15 million in 1995 to 23.8 million in 2000, or 16.5% of all workers. By 2004, more than 35 million had used the FMLA. As illustrated in Table 1, there were percentage increases in all of the categories except for taking time off for one's own health. Most relevant to this discussion, however, was an increase in the percentage of workers who took leave to care for an ill elderly parent, rising from 8.6% in 1995, to 13% in 2000. In absolute numbers, it represented an increase from 1.3 million caring for an elderly parent in 1995

TABLE 1. Percentage of All Leave-Takers Reporting Reasons

	1995 Survey	2000 Survey
Own health	60.0%	52.4%
Care for newborn, adopted or foster child	13.3%	18.5%
Care for ill parent	8.6%	13.0%
Care for ill child	7.6%	11.5%
Maternity/disability	3.8%	7.9%
Care for ill spouse	3.7%	6.4%
Care for ill relative	3.1%	NA

Note: Percentages do not add up to 100% because respondents could select more than one category.
Source: Author's interpretation of data provided by the U.S. Department of Labor, 2000.

to 3.1 million in 2000. Based on demographic projections, this increase in elder care under the FMLA is likely to continue well into the future.

THE ROLE OF THE FAMILY IN LONG-TERM CARE

The number of persons aged 65 and older has increased substantially over the last 30 years (Manton & Stallard, 1994). Just in the 10-year period between 1980 and 1990, the number of persons 65 or older increased from 25.5 million (11.3% of the total U.S. population) to 31 million (12.5% of the total population). Equally significant is the trend within the trend. That is, during that same time period, the population of those over 85 grew considerably, from 2.2 million in 1980 (about 1% of the U.S. population) to 3.0 million in 1990 (about 1.2% of the U.S. population) (U.S. Bureau of the Census, 1996). This growing age group in particular, with its multiple chronic illnesses, will place great demands on the health care system in general and family caregivers in particular (Wisensale, 1999).

According to existing census data, moderate projections indicate that the population of people 65 and over who represented 12.5% of the total U.S. population in 1990 will increase to 13.3% by 2010 and reach as high as 20.4% by 2050. For the elderly minority, the increase is even more rapid, rising from 13% of the elderly population in 1990 to 16% in 2000, to 22% in 2020, and to 33% by 2050 (U.S. Bureau of the Census, 1996). Clearly, with the baby-boom population aging, the demand for family care will increase, and companies will be pressured by employees for release time to assist aging parents.

According to a recent study by the Families and Work Institute (1997), more than one-third (35%) of American workers had significant elder care responsibilities in the previous year. Further, more than a third of employees with elder care obligations had to reduce their workload or take time off to provide family care. This finding coincides with a 1997 study of 1,509 people conducted for Metropolitan Life by the National Alliance for Caregivers and the American Association for Retired Persons (MetLife Study, 1997). Surveyors found that one in four families had at least one adult who had provided care for an elderly relative or friend in the previous 12 months. However, only 23% of companies with 100 or more employees have programs in place to support elder care (Families and Work Institute, 1997). "Elder care is to the twenty-first century what child care has been the last few decades," contends Joyce Ruddock, head of the Long-Term Care Group at Metropolitan Life (*New York Times*, 1999: 1).

THE ISSUE OF COST IN LONG-TERM CARE

Long-term care is extremely expensive for the elderly, their families, and American taxpayers. In order to understand this complex issue, at least four points should be emphasized. First, Medicare does not cover long-term care (other than for a short transition period), either in nursing homes or at home (Binstock, Cluff, & Von Mering, 1996). Medicaid, on the other hand, is available for such coverage, but it is means-tested and, therefore, limited to low-income elderly. Still, between 60 and 80% of Medicaid funds are consumed by the elderly for long-term care services–either for institutional or home care (Weiner, 1996). Second, long-term care insurance, once viewed as a potential cure-all for the long-term care crisis, is not only expensive but also limited in scope. At least two studies report that only 20% of the aged population can afford private long-term care insurance, and far fewer elect to purchase it (Crown, Capitman, & Leutz, 1992) (Weiner, Illston, & Hanley, 1994). Third, long-term care spending is still biased toward institutional care, with only six states spending less than half their total long-term expenditures on institutional care (MEDSTAT Group Inc., 2002). Still, there is much variation among states. For example, in 2002 Louisiana devoted 90% of its long-term care expenditures to institutional care and only 10% to home care. Oregon, on the other hand, spent only 27% on institutional care compared to 73% on home care (MEDSTAT Group Inc., 2002). And fourth, out-of-pocket expenses are high. It is estimated that about 44% of the total costs of long-term care is covered by families (Weiner, Illston, & Hanley, 1994). Similarly, out-of-pocket payments cover 51% of nursing home costs and 26% of home care expenditures (Feinberg, 1997).

According to the National Academy on Aging (2000), uncompensated care provided by family members and friends was estimated to have an economic value of $196 billion in 1997. This amount far exceeds the total spent that year on nursing home care ($83 billion) and home health care ($32 billion) (Levine & Memmott, 1999). Unpaid family care saves taxpayers billions of dollars annually. For those who are paid, however, 43% receive payments from Medicaid, and about 37% of paid caregivers receive out-of-pocket payments from the elderly who employ them (National Academy on Aging, 2000).

But the money saved for taxpayers by the gallant efforts of family caregivers does not come without cost to someone. Nor should it be assumed that such care will continue without disruption. According to the "MetLife Juggling Act Study," caregiving costs individuals as much as $659,000 over their lifetimes in wages lost, and Social Security and pension contributions not being made because they "take time off, leave their jobs entirely, or experience compromised opportunities for training, promotions, and 'plum' assignments" (MetLife Study, 1999: 1).

Broken down further, the caregivers studied reported $566,500 in lost wages, $67,000 in lost retirement contributions, and $25,500 in lost Social Security benefits. Added to these figures was an additional $19,500 in food costs, transportation expenses, assistance with rents and mortgages, and the cost to retain home care professionals. Furthermore, nearly 30% stated they had passed on promotions, training opportunities, and new assignments. About 84% of the caregivers made adjustments to their work schedules by taking sick leave or vacation time if available, decreasing work hours and thus reducing their income, taking an unpaid leave of absence, switching from full- to part-time employment, and resigning or retiring. Equally important, it was learned that few of the respondents' employers offered programs, resources, or services to assist their employees in meeting their caregiving obligations (MetLife Study, 1999).

Policymakers in Washington were not oblivious to the toll that caretaking responsibilities were taking on America's families, both emotionally and financially, having adopted the National Family Caregiver Support Program, the Dependent Care Tax Credit that included coverage of elder care, and permitted waivers that provided direct payment to caregivers under Medicaid. (For more information on the National Family Caregivers Support Program, see "Preliminary Experiences of the States in Implementing the National Family Caregiver Support Program: A 50-State Study" in this volume.) Nor were legislators unaware of the weaknesses of the original Family and Medical Leave Act. Between 1993 and 1999, almost 20 initiatives were put forth by members of Congress to expand the Family and Medical Leave Act. Some wanted the law to apply to smaller companies; others wanted to include additional hours to address basic family needs, such as taking children to dental appointments or for attending parent-teacher meetings. Still others proposed that the coverage be expanded to include domestic partners, parents-in-law, and grandparents (Gladstone, 1999; Jordan, 1999). In the meantime, a new White House strategy was slowly emerging.

TOWARD PAID LEAVE:
THE DEVOLUTION OF THE FMLA AND STATE STRATEGIES

In his commencement address at Grambling State University in Louisiana on May 23, 1999, President Clinton announced two new initiatives aimed at the FMLA. First, he directed the Department of Labor to explore ways states may use surplus unemployment insurance funds to subsidize parents who use the FMLA to care for a newborn or newly adopted child (thus "Baby UI"). The second initiative recommended that federal employees be permitted to use up to twelve weeks of accrued sick leave to care for a seriously ill child, parent, or spouse. Prior to 1999, federal workers could only use up to 13 days of accrued sick leave per year to care for seriously ill family members. "I believe it is imperative that your country give you the tools to succeed not only in the workplace but also at home. If you or any American has to choose between being a good parent and successful in your careers, you have paid a terrible price, and so has your country," he told the graduates (President's Commencement Address, 1999).

The following day, Clinton issued an Executive Memorandum entitled "New Tools to Help Parents Balance Work and Family." In the memo, the President ordered the Secretary of Labor, Alexis Herman, to propose regulations that would allow states to use Unemployment Insurance (UI) funds to support parents on leave following the birth or adoption of a child. He also called upon the secretary to develop model legislation that states could adopt in following these new regulations (Presidential Memorandum, 1999).

Under the president's proposal, states were permitted to tap the surpluses of their Unemployment Insurance trust funds to cover 12 weeks of parental leave. In short, any employee leaving work under the FMLA for the birth or adoption of a child would be classified as temporarily laid off, and therefore declared eligible for unemployment compensation. The idea runs parallel to the use of Temporary Disability Insurance (TDI), which provides a wage replacement for new mothers in five states (New York, New Jersey, Rhode Island, California, and Hawaii). Companies in TDI states are required to offer paid leave to new mothers, just as it would be offered to other employees who are ill or temporarily disabled (Meyers, 1995).

Spurred on by Clinton's initiative, 13 states, between May 23, 1999, and July 2000, introduced legislation that included a provision for some type of paid family leave. These included California, Connecticut, Georgia, Illinois, Indiana, Maine, Massachusetts, Maryland, Minnesota, New Hampshire, New Jersey, Vermont, and Washington. No state succeeded in passing paid leave legislation, and only three states (Connecticut, Massachusetts, and New Jersey) proposed coverage that extended beyond "baby care" (Baby UI) and included elder care. Connecticut's proposal, for example, was designed to use only UI funds to cover the birth or adoption of a child while other leaves, such as time off for elder care, would be funded through a new Medical Leave Insurance Fund. Both Massachusetts and New Jersey produced similar hybrid proposals that would allow UI to cover childbirth and adoption, but care of other family members would be funded through separate mechanisms.

One year later, in 2001, the number of states proposing paid leave doubled from 13 to 26. A summary of the state initiatives is presented in Table 2. Although there was much activity in the states, no state succeeded in passing paid-leave legislation until California succeeded in 2002. And, as presented in Table 2, only five of the 26 states included coverage of elder care in their legislative initiatives: Hawaii, Indiana, Massachusetts, New Hampshire, and New Jersey. All five states produced a variety of proposals that ranged from exclusive use of UI benefits (Indiana) to the use of UI and TDI hybrid models (Massachusetts and New Jersey), to the creation of trust funds independent of either TDI or UI models (Hawaii and New Hampshire). But the most important point to be emphasized here is that apparently relatively few states are willing to support caregivers of the elderly, despite demographic trends that reveal a growing elderly population and a rise in dual-earner couples.

RECENT TRENDS AND POLICY INITIATIVES

On October 9, 2003, George W. Bush rescinded Clinton's executive order that permitted states to use UI trust funds for covering paid leave. Almost immediately, the UI model was abandoned and states shifted their attention to sick leave as a means for providing paid family care. Specifically, states have put forth initiatives that have a twofold purpose: to allow employees to use their six days to care for ailing family members and to increase the number of sick days available. On average, those who have paid sick leave coverage are allotted only about 14 days a year.

According to the National Partnership for Women and Families (2004), 48 states have laws or regulations allowing public employees to

TABLE 2. State Paid Leave Initiatives–2001-2003

State	Proposal
Arizona	Up to 12 weeks of UI for care of newborn or newly adopted child
California**	Recommended expanding TDI to cover family care (elder care)
Connecticut	Motion to permit public employees to use sick leave for child care
Florida	Up to 12 weeks of UI to care for a newborn or newly adopted child
Hawaii *	"Family Leave Insurance Fund" would cover family care
Illinois	12 weeks of UI coverage for childbirth or newly adopted child
Indiana *	12 weeks of UI coverage to care for ill family member
Iowa	Accrued sick leave to be used for the adoption of a child
Kansas	12 weeks of UI coverage to care for newborn or adopted child
Maryland	12 weeks of UI to care for newborn or newly adopted child
Massachusetts *	UI coverage for parental leave, TDI coverage for family care
Minnesota	UI coverage for newborn/adopted child (state shares costs)
Mississippi	12 weeks of UI coverage for birth or adoption of a child
Missouri	Tax credits for employers who provide paid maternity leave
Nebraska	12 weeks of UI coverage for newborn or newly adopted child
New Hampshire *	Payroll tax to fund a "Family and Disability Trust Fund"
New Jersey *	TDI/UI hybrid to cover newborn, adoption, or family care
New Mexico	12 weeks of UI coverage for newborn or newly adopted child
New York	Effort to expand TDI to cover family care (ongoing study)
Oregon	12 weeks of UI coverage for newborn or newly adopted child
Pennsylvania	Revised 2000 bill that covered newborns and adoptees
Texas	12 weeks of leave under UI for childbirth and newly adopted child
Vermont	Use of general funds to cover parental leave–not UI funded
Virginia	Study completed in 2000 recommended paid leave under FMLA
Washington	"Family Leave Insurance Fund" funded by workers and employers
Wisconsin	Several proposals designed to provide a wage replacement

*Indicates coverage for elder care
**Indicates paid leave and coverage for elder care
Source: Author's interpretation of data provided by the National Partnership for Women and Families, 2004.

use sick leave to care for sick family members, with much variation in the definition of "family members." Only three states require private employers to provide sick leave for their workers. Consequently, about half (47%) of private sector workers, and 59 million total workers in the United States, have no paid sick days at all. There are 86 million workers in the United States who do not have a single paid sick day that can be used to care for sick children, not to mention care of the elderly (Lovell, 2004).

With no federal law that guarantees sick leave to all workers, the United States stands in sharp contrast to other nations. Of the 139 nations that provide paid leave for short- or long-term illnesses, 117 countries guarantee their workers a week or more of paid sick days per year (National Partnership, 2004). In short, if the strategy of paid-leave advocates is to "piggy-back" existing sick leave policies in the states, it may be shortsighted with respect to long-term care of the elderly for at least two reasons: (1) Half the workers are not covered by sick leave policies. (2) The number of sick days allocated are relatively few, averaging about 14 days per year. Elder care demands tend to be sporadic and often last longer than two weeks.

One success story for paid-leave advocates took place in 2002. California, by expanding its state disability insurance program from maternal to family care, became the first and only state to adopt a comprehensive paid family and medical leave insurance policy. Workers can receive a partial wage replacement (55%-60% of wages) with a cap during six weeks of leave per year to care for a newborn, newly adopted or foster child, or to care for a seriously ill family member, *including an elderly parent* and a domestic partner. Funded solely by employee contributions, the average annual cost per worker is about $27.

Meanwhile, in the summer of 2004, Senator Edward M. Kennedy (D-MA) and Representative Rosa L. DeLauro (D-CT) introduced the Healthy Families Act, which would guarantee seven paid sick days a year to full-time workers. Workers in any private company or governmental unit with at least 15 employees would be covered and, therefore, be able to take time off for one's own illness or to care for a family member. However, there has been little movement on the proposed bill so far.

ADDRESSING WEAKNESSES
AND MAKING POLICY RECOMMENDATIONS

The passage of the National Family Caregiver Support Program (NFCSP) under the Older Americans Act Amendments of 2000 is "the first federally-funded program implemented at the state level designed specifically to support the service needs of family caregivers of older people" (Feinberg & Newman, 2004: 760). This act coincides with recent studies that revealed a growing demand among caregivers for more government support (Silverstein & Parrott, 2001). An important policy objective in most states is to create and maintain a balanced long-term care system that includes a variety of home- and community-based support services (Weiner, Tilly, & Alecxih, 2002). A key component of this strategy should be the expansion of leave policy by providing a wage replacement and guaranteeing that caregivers of the elderly be included. To this end, the following recommendations are suggested.

There are at least four steps that can be taken to make the Family and Medical Leave Act more compatible with the demands associated with long-term care of the aged. First, let us make family leave paid leave and do it immediately! As discussed earlier, dual-earner couples and single parents are especially burdened financially–despite the recent economic boom. Of the two industrialized nations in the world without paid leave, the United States is richer and stronger. It has taken us much too long as a nation to recognize and respect housework and caregiving responsibilities as *work*. Therefore, particularly in light of a growing elderly population, it is time for such activities to be compensated. Caregivers will continue to provide services, save taxpayers money on institutional care while remaining attached to the labor force. Corporations, families, and society in general will be better for it.

Second, in pushing for paid leave, many states dropped the intergenerational component of the original bill. That is, in 1985, when legislative strategists deliberately expanded the original bill to include family care, they did so for two reasons: (1) They were fostering "equal treatment" (family care) over "special treatment" (maternity leave). (2) A broader-based bill that extended beyond maternity leave attracted more votes in the House and Senate, giving a shot in the arm to a fledgling coalition that was dividing its time between lobbying for child care (passed in 1990) on one hand and family leave on the other (adopted in 1993). It does not necessarily follow that advocates should now shrink the benefit by confining it only to care of newborns in order to appease opponents and attract political support. But the "Baby UI" initiatives did precisely that, and the current push to retrofit employees' sick leave as a means of providing paid leave will do little to address the needs of caregivers of the elderly.

The facts are clear. We are about to witness the retirement of the baby boomers. The state will depend on informal family care to help cushion the costs of what certainly will be an astronomically expensive long-term care system. Requests for intermittent leave to care for an elderly parent will increase substantially. Furthermore, by maintaining *family* in the policy and not specifically targeting childbirth, the growing backlash among childless workers is more likely to be defused. After all, it is quite likely that at some point those workers too will need time off to care for a spouse, a parent, or themselves. And besides, by offering paid leave only under circumstances associated with childbirth, are we not trading in "equal treatment" for "special treatment" and revisiting a familiar battleground from years past?

Third, family leave should apply to more companies and be available to more workers. The 50-worker threshold should immediately be reduced to at least 25, and lowered regularly over time so that more employees in smaller companies are covered under the law. As discussed previously, those in higher-income brackets who work for larger firms are more likely to take leave than are lower-income employees in smaller companies. Most of the potential caregivers are women (much more family care needs to be done by men) who tend to work for lower wages in smaller businesses. Not only do they deserve the same level of benefits as those who earn more in bigger companies, but it is also in society's best interest that they be rewarded. They will remain attached to the workforce and provide an important service (caregiving) to society.

Fourth, the law should be further expanded in another way. As currently written, it is insensitive to changing family patterns. For example, grandparent care, in-law care, and the care provided by partners in a committed, domestic-partnership type of relationship are not covered. A few states, such as California, have addressed several of these shortcomings; other states and the federal government should follow. Clearly, the family has changed and continues to do so. Unfortunately, too many well-meaning policymakers continue to harbor nostalgic images of the family that are anchored in 1950 TV sitcoms. If we expect to address our future long-term care needs adequately, we need to recognize and value families more for the functions they perform than for the forms they take.

AUTHOR NOTE

Steven K. Wisensale, PhD, is Professor of Public Policy in the School of Family Studies at the University of Connecticut. His research and teaching interests include family policy, work and family issues, and aging policy. He is the author of *Family Leave Policy: The Political Economy of Work and Family in America* (2001). Professor Wisensale can be contacted at The School of Family Studies, U-2058, University of Connecticut, Storrs, CT 06269 (E-mail: Steven.Wisensale@Uconn.edu).

REFERENCES

Binstock, R., Cluff, L., & Von Mering, O. (1996). Issues affecting the future of long-term care. In R. Binstock, L. Cluff, and O. von Mering (Eds), *The future of long-term care: Social and policy issues*. Baltimore, MD: Johns Hopkins University Press.

Commission on Leave (1996). *A workable balance: Report to congress on family and medical leave policies*. Washington, DC: U.S. Department of Labor.

Crown, W., Capitman, J., & Leutz, W. (1992). Economic rationality, the affordability of private long-term care insurance, and the role for public policy. *The Gerontologist, 32:* 478-85.

Families and Work Institute (1997). *National study of the changing workforce.* New York: Families and Work Institute.

Feinberg, L., & Newman, S. (2004). A study of 10 states since passage of the national family caregiver support program: Policies, perceptions, and program development. *The Gerontologist, 44*(6): 760-769.

Feinberg, L. (1997). *Options for supporting informal and family caregiving: A policy paper.* San Francisco: American Society on Aging.

Gladstone, L. (1999). The Family and Medical Leave Act: Proposed amendments. Order code: 97017. Washington, DC: Congressional Research Services.

Jordan, L. (1999). FMLA proposals. Office of Legislative Research. Hartford, CT: Connecticut General Assembly.

Levine, A., & Memmott, M. (1999). The economic value of informal caregiving. *Health Affairs, 18*(2): 182-188.

Lovell, V. (2004). *No time to be sick: Why everyone suffers when workers don't have paid leave.* Washington, DC: Institute for Women's Policy Research.

Manton, K., & Stallard, E. (1994). Interaction of disability dynamics and mortality. In L. Martin and S. Preston (Eds.), *Demography of aging,* 217-278. Committee on Population, National Research Council. Washington, DC: National Academy Press.

MEDSTAT Group Inc. (2002). The long-term care tab. Ann Arbor, MI: MEDSTAT Group Inc.

MetLife (1997). MetLife study of employer costs for working caregivers. Westport, CT: MetLife Mature Market Institute.

MetLife (1999). MetLife juggling act study. Westport, CT: MetLife Mature Market Institute.

Meyers, M. (1995). Taking pregnancy leaves. Minneapolis: *Star Tribune,* February 6, 1995: A1.

National Academy on an Aging Society (2000). *Caregiving: Helping the elderly with activity limitations.* Washington, DC: National Academy on an Aging Society.

National Partnership (2004). *Get well soon: Americans can't afford to be sick.* Washington, DC: National Partnership for Women and Families.

New York Times (1999). What's the problem? Week in Review, August 9, 1999.

President's Commencement Address (1999). Grambling State University, Grambling, LA, May 23. Washington, DC: The White House.

Presidential Memorandum (1999). Memorandum for the heads of executive departments and agencies: New tools to help parents balance work and family. May 24, 1999. Washington, DC: The White House.

Silverstein, M., & Parrott, T. (2001). Attitudes toward government policies that assist informal caregivers. *Research on Aging, 23*(3): 349-374.

U.S. Bureau of the Census (1996). *65 + in the United States.* Current Population Reports, Special Studies, P23-190. Washington, DC: United States Bureau of the Census.

U.S. Department of Labor (2000). *Balancing the needs of families and employers: Family and medical leave surveys.* Washington, DC: U.S. Department of Labor.

Weiner, J. (1996). *Can Medicaid long-term care expenditures for the elderly be reduced?* New York: The Commonwealth Fund.

Wiener, J., Illston, L., & Hanley, R. (1994). *Sharing the burden: Strategies for public and private long-term care insurance.* Washington, DC: Brookings Institution.

Weiner, J., Tilly, J., & Alecxih, L. (2002). Home and community-based services in seven states. *Health Care Financing Review, 23*: 89-114.

Wisensale, S. (2001). *Family leave policy: The Political Economy of Work and Family in America.* Armonk, NY: M. E. Sharpe.

Wisensale, S. (1999). Grappling with the generational equity debate: An ongoing challenge for the public administrator. *Public Integrity, 1*: 1-19.

doi:10.1300/J031v18n03_06

Preliminary Experiences of the States in Implementing the National Family Caregiver Support Program: A 50-State Study

Lynn Friss Feinberg, MSW
Sandra L. Newman, MPH

National Center on Caregiving, Family Caregiver Alliance

SUMMARY. Despite increased attention to policy choices to support family and informal caregivers, relatively little is known about states' experiences in providing caregiver support services. This article reports on the first nationwide survey of all 50 states and the District of Columbia in providing caregiver services since the passage of the National Family Caregiver Support Program. State program administrators reported that their program differs from other home and community-based services because of the explicit focus on the family or informal caregiver. Results suggest that despite an increasing availability of caregiver supports in all 50 states, there is also a great unevenness in services and service options for family caregivers across the states and within states. doi:10.1300/J031v18n03_07 *[Article copies available for a fee from The Haworth Document Delivery Service: 1-800-HAWORTH. E-mail address: <docdelivery@haworthpress.com> Website: <http://www.HaworthPress.com> © 2006 by The Haworth Press, Inc. All rights reserved.]*

KEYWORDS. Family care, consumer direction, state policy, home and community-based care

[Haworth co-indexing entry note]: "Preliminary Experiences of the States in Implementing the National Family Caregiver Support Program: A 50-State Study." Feinberg, Lynn Friss, and Sandra L. Newman. Co-published simultaneously in *Journal of Aging & Social Policy* (The Haworth Press, Inc.) Vol. 18, No. 3/4, 2006, pp. 95-113; and: *Family and Aging Policy* (ed: Francis G. Caro) The Haworth Press, Inc., 2006, pp. 95-113. Single or multiple copies of this article are available for a fee from The Haworth Document Delivery Service [1-800-HAWORTH, 9:00 a.m. - 5:00 p.m. (EST). E-mail address: docdelivery@haworthpress.com].

Available online at http://jasp.haworthpress.com
© 2006 by The Haworth Press, Inc. All rights reserved.
doi:10.1300/J031v18n03_07

INTRODUCTION

The need to strengthen family and informal caregivers, and to recognize their public rights to their own supports, is a central issue in our aging society. The vast majority (78%) of adults in the United States who receive long-term care at home get all care exclusively from unpaid family and friends, mostly wives and adult daughters. Another 14% receive some combination of family care and paid assistance; only 8% rely on formal care alone (Thompson, 2004). Indeed, the importance of the family's role in long-term care is mounting because of the policy shift away from institutional care and toward more home and community-based care. In recent years, demands on family caregivers to locate, access, coordinate, and provide everyday care have grown due to advances in medical technology, changes in our health care delivery system, shortages in the direct care workforce, and an increasingly fragmented and confusing home and community-based services (HCBS) system. At both the federal and state levels, debate has intensified about policy choices to support family and informal care and to improve the capacity of family and friends to provide such care.

Although family members often undertake caregiving willingly and find it a source of great personal satisfaction, they need support services themselves because they oftentimes face substantial emotional, physical, and financial problems as a result of caring for someone with a chronic illness or disability (Aneshensel, Pearlin, Mullan, Zarit, & Whitlatch, 1995; Schultz et al., 1997). One recent study of the long-term effects of caregiving on women's economic well-being found that caregiving for a parent substantially increased women's risks of living in poverty and receiving public assistance in later life (Wakabayashi & Donato, 2004). As Levine (2004) has noted, "The problem is not that public policy looks first to families but that it generally looks only to families and fails to support those who accept responsibility" (p. 103).

In 2000, Congress authorized a new program under the federal Older Americans Act explicitly to assist family caregivers of older people, known as the National Family Caregiver Support Program (NFCSP). With its creation, family and informal caregivers are now recognized as consumers in their own right. However, little is known about states' experiences in providing caregiver support since the passage of the NFCSP. This research is the first to examine caregiver programs in all 50 states and the District of Columbia funded under the NFCSP.

BACKGROUND

States approach the design of HCBS programs, including those to support caregivers, in different ways. Some states view caregiver support as part of their programs that serve frail elders or adults with disabilities. Others see caregiver support as a separate program with distinct eligibility criteria; they seek to ensure the explicit recognition of family and informal caregivers as individuals with rights to their own services and supports (Feinberg, Newman, Gray, Kolb, & Fox-Grage, 2004).

Before passage of the NFCSP in 2000, state general revenues financed most publicly funded caregiver services. However, some states have covered respite care, an important benefit for family caregivers, under their Medicaid HCBS waiver programs. Today, the NFCSP, state-funded programs and Medicaid waivers provide the bulk of public financing for family caregiving.

National Family Caregiver Support Program (NFCSP)

To date, the enactment of the NFCSP stands as the federal government's most significant recognition of and commitment to providing direct services to caregivers. Under broad federal guidelines, the NFCSP calls for the states, working in partnership with area agencies on aging (AAAs) and local service providers, to develop multifaceted systems of support for family and informal caregivers within five basic service categories: (1) information to caregivers about available services; (2) assistance to caregivers in gaining access to supportive services; (3) individual counseling, support groups and caregiver training; (4) respite care; and (5) supplemental services (e.g., emergency response systems, home modifications), on a limited basis, to complement the care provided by caregivers.

The NFCSP was developed as an initial effort to begin to address the service needs of a segment of the caregiver population. Congress appropriated $125 million in fiscal year 2001, $141.5 million in fiscal year 2002, and $155.2 million for the NFCSP in fiscal year 2003, the year of this study. This modest funding is consistent with the historic pattern of funding for the various service programs under the Older Americans Act. For fiscal year 2003, NFCSP formula grants to the states totaled $138.7 million, ranging from a high of $13.8 million in California to a low of $705,756 in eleven states (Alaska, Delaware, Hawaii, Idaho, Montana, New Hampshire, North Dakota, Rhode Island, South Dakota,

Vermont, and Wyoming) and the District of Columbia. Another portion of the funds, approximately $6.2 million in fiscal year 2003, supported grants to Indian Tribal Organizations. Funds in the amount of $7.5 million have also supported a National Innovations Program, the goal of which has been to conduct activities of national significance.

The federal government gives states considerable discretion in the design and administration of the NFCSP. Under the new program, states use federal funds to offer direct support services to family caregivers of persons age 60 and older. States can also reserve up to a maximum of 10% of their funding to provide support services to grandparents and relative caregivers of children age 18 and younger. All income groups are eligible for services, but states must give priority to those providing care to older individuals in the greatest social or economic need with particular attention to low-income individuals and older relatives caring for children with mental retardation/developmental disabilities. Functional eligibility criteria vary by type of service: individuals 60 years and older must have two or more limitations in activities of daily living (ADLs) or a cognitive impairment for the caregiver to be eligible for respite or supplemental services. Other service categories (e.g., counseling, support groups) are available to family caregivers regardless of the care receiver's functional status.

The implementation of the new NFCSP takes place within an emerging policy direction in states to address support to family caregivers. The federal government's New Freedom Initiative, established by executive order in 2001, outlines a plan to assist states and local communities in responding to the U.S. Supreme Court's decision in *Olmstead v. L.C.* In this landmark decision, the Court ruled that states must provide services in community, rather than institutional, settings for certain persons with disabilities who receive assistance in publicly funded programs. The New Freedom Initiative identifies lack of family support as a major barrier to community living for persons with disabilities, underscoring the need for greater assistance to informal caregivers (Department of Health and Human Services [DHHS], 2002).

PURPOSE OF THE STUDY

The present research is a descriptive study, the first to characterize and analyze the preliminary experiences of all 50 states and the District of Columbia in providing caregiver support services under the Older

Americans Act's NFCSP. The larger, two-year research project from which the present study is drawn examined a broad range of federal and state-funded programs that provide some component of caregiver support services in each of the 50 states and across states, focusing on state agencies responsible for the administration of the NFCSP, Aged/Disabled Medicaid waiver programs, and state-funded programs (Feinberg et al., 2004). In this article, five policy areas are addressed: program development; eligibility and assessment; services and access; consumer direction; and systems development. These policy areas are framed around the following key questions: (1) How did the infusion of federal funds through the NFCSP enable states to provide support services to family caregivers? (2) Who is considered the client population in the program? (3) What approaches are states taking to assess the needs of family and informal caregivers? (4) What services do states provide under the NFCSP and how do families access them? (5) What is the role of consumer direction in the NFCSP? (6) How do states view issues around the integration of caregiver support into HCBS? (7) What are the main challenges faced by states in implementing services under the NFCSP?

METHODS

This study used the survey method, with written surveys and telephone interviews, to collect the programmatic information. Data were collected for fiscal year 2003. Respondents were NFCSP state administrators in the 50 states and the District of Columbia ($N = 51$).

The term "family caregiver" was used to include care provided by relatives, friends, or neighbors to persons 60 years or older or adults (age 18-59) with physical and/or adult-onset cognitive disabilities (e.g., traumatic brain injury). These persons could be primary or secondary caregivers, provide full- or part-time help, and could live with the person being cared for or live separately.

This study did not attempt to detail all the eligible populations under the NFCSP. Consequently, this study did not examine the Native American Caregiver Support Program, caregiver support for persons with developmental disabilities, or grandparents raising grandchildren. These programs are important to family caregivers and people with disabilities, but beyond the scope of this research.

Data Collection

Survey development was guided by a national advisory committee of experts in the field, stakeholders, and previous state studies conducted by the authors. Data were collected in two parts. First, a cover letter and the written (Part 1) survey were sent to SUA directors and key contacts, usually the state program administrator of the NFCSP. The written survey was also sent via email with hyperlink access to the Web-based survey instrument. More than half (59%) of the 51 NFCSP respondents utilized the electronic format. Following receipt of the Part 1 survey, semi-structured telephone interviews (Part 2) were conducted with state respondents by research staff. Parts 1 and 2 of the 50-state survey were pre-tested with state administrators in Alabama and Hawaii. Follow-up calls to the state respondents were made, when necessary, to clarify data or responses. Copies of the instruments are available from the authors.

Part 1 was a written survey that included 30 questions, 29 fixed-choice and one open-ended. Questions addressed program background, program eligibility/assessment process, program administration, services, consumer direction, systems development, and other issues. Part 2 was a semi-structured telephone interview and included 17 questions of which three were fixed-choice and 14 were open-ended. The Part 2 interview included questions about the caregiver program specifically, and gathered impressions about family caregivers within the state, and about the state's system of HCBS generally. The telephone interview lasted, on average, 34 minutes. All (100%) state NFCSPs participated in Parts 1 and 2 of the study.

Analysis

Part 1 data were analyzed using SPSS for Windows, version 11.0. Descriptive statistics, including frequency distributions and cross-tabulations of selected questions, were used to characterize closed-ended questions. The project team developed a set of codes to analyze questions with open-ended responses. For the Part 2 telephone interviews, a qualitative, grounded-theory (Glaser & Strauss, 1967) approach was used throughout the analysis. Frequencies were calculated by program type and for the entire sample.

RESULTS

Program Development

The infusion of federal funds under the NFCSP enabled more than one in three (36%) states to provide some direct support to informal caregivers of older people for the first time (see Figure 1). Before the enactment of the NFCSP in 2000, 18 states and the District of Columbia had no state program primarily funded through state general funds that served family or informal caregivers, neither a caregiver-specific state-wide program (e.g., California's Caregiver Resource Centers) nor a caregiver component within a broader HCBS program (e.g., North Dakota's Family Home Care Program). As part of the larger study, we identified 50 state-funded programs in 32 states providing some support for family or informal caregivers that had predated the NFCSP. Often, these programs were part of state-funded HCBS where one or more service components (e.g., respite care) indirectly helped family caregivers, although the programs themselves targeted services to either frail elders or adults with physical and/or adult-onset cognitive disabilities, such as

FIGURE 1. Caregiver Support Programs in the States Prior to Passage of the NFCSP, 2000

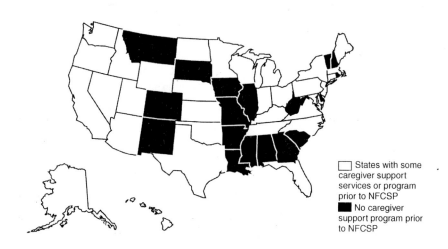

☐ States with some caregiver support services or program prior to NFCSP
■ No caregiver support program prior to NFCSP

Note: Figure is based on the State of the States in Family Caregiver Support Survey (Part 1, Question 4), National Center on Caregiving, Family Caregiver Alliance, San Francisco, CA, 2004.

Alzheimer's disease. In only a few states (e.g., California, New Jersey, Pennsylvania, Wisconsin) has caregiver support had a long tradition; in these states, state-funded programs have historically supported family caregivers through state legislative mandates that provide explicit recognition of the need to support caregivers.

Eligibility and Assessment

A program's client designation impacts eligibility and shapes how program services are configured and delivered. We asked respondents, "Who is considered the client in this program?" Nearly three-fourths (73%) of the state administrators (36 states and the District of Columbia) identified the caregiver as the primary client in the NFCSP program, in keeping with the new mandate under the Older Americans Act to provide explicit support services to family and informal caregivers of older persons. Another 26% or 13 states viewed both the caregiver and care receiver (i.e., older person) as the primary client group, taking a more "family systems" approach to eligibility and service delivery. Only one state NFCSP respondent considered the older person to be the client in the family caregiver support program. *"I think we 'get' it now,"* said one state NFCSP administrator, *"but that was one of the biggest challenges and one of the lessons learned. The focus [of the program] is the caregiver, the client is the caregiver, and the recipient is the caregiver too. That is quite a switch from how we think, especially in the HCBS world."*

The aim of an assessment is to identify needs for support and assistance and to serve as a basis for a plan of care. Although virtually all state HCBS programs use some type of an assessment tool to determine the functional level and unmet needs of the care receiver, few uniformly assess the caregiver's well-being and his or her own support needs even though understanding the role, multiple stressors, and the particular situation of the family caregiver is essential to any care plan developed for the care receiver. While the NFCSP provides distinct support services for caregivers, it includes no mandate for caregiver assessment.

In this study, the great majority (82%) of 51 NFCSP respondents reported that they assessed the needs and situation, in some way, of both the older adult and the family caregiver. The majority of these state program administrators (69%) viewed family caregivers as their client population, although they recognized the importance of collecting information on both members of the dyad to improve outcomes. Nearly one-third (31%) of the remaining NFCSP programs considered both members of the dyad (i.e., the care receiver and the family caregiver) to be the program client and reported that they assessed the needs of both. Another 10% of the NFCSPs (5 states) assessed only the needs of the family caregiver, and 8% (4 states) reported assessments of the older person only.

Although virtually all (92%) of the 51 NFCSPs reported assessing the needs of the family caregiver or conducting dual assessments of the caregiver and care receiver in some fashion, only 41% (21 states and the District of Columbia) reported that their state programs used a uniform assessment tool to assess caregiver needs. Moreover, the types of information collected were found to vary from state to state under the NFCSP. When the state NFCSP administrators who utilized a uniform assessment tool in their program (21 states and the District of Columbia) were asked to identify the areas covered in a caregiver assessment from a closed list of nine domains, the top five most often cited areas of assessment were the caregiver's ability to provide care (76%); basic demographic information, such as age or gender (71%); caregiver strain, (67%); and care frequency, caregiver physical health, and caregiver depression (57% each).

Despite varying approaches to assessment across and within states, there was broad consensus among the NFCSP respondents that caregiver assessment issues were a main topic of interest and program support need. Virtually all (92%) of the NFCSP program administrators either "strongly agreed" or "agreed" that technical assistance or training on caregiver assessment issues would assist staff to address caregiver needs more effectively within their states.

Services and Access

With overall guidance provided by the Administration on Aging, the NFCSP is designed to offer a broad range of services and service options, and to offer flexibility to the states to develop and deliver services that best meet caregiver needs within five basic service categories. *Information* to caregivers about available services includes individual and group information activities, such as public education and outreach at health fairs. *Assistance* in helping caregivers gain access to the services and resources available within their community includes consultations that assist caregivers with decision making. *Individual counseling, support groups and caregiver training* offer families help in making decisions and solving problems related to their caregiving roles. *Respite care* includes a range of strategies and approaches to provide temporary relief for caregivers from their care responsibilities by providing short-term help to the care receiver. *Supplemental services* are any other services, as defined by the state, to support caregivers (e.g., emergency response systems). These services are to be offered on a limited basis, with no more than 20% of the NFCSP funds to be used for this service category.

We asked state NFCSP administrators to identify the services that their program provides specifically to family caregivers from a closed list of 20 items. As shown in Table 1, the state NFCSPs offer a broad array of caregiver support services. Respite care was found to top the list, and is now provided, to some degree, by all caregiver programs in the 50 states and the District of Columbia. A range of other key support services are also offered by the states, including caregiver education and training (94% of NFCSPs); support groups (90%); family consultations and care management (84%); individual and/or family counseling (80%); purchase of consumable supplies (67%); legal/financial consultations (61%); family meetings (43%); cash grants to purchase goods or services (24%); and eHealth applications (12%).

Respite care addresses a pressing need identified by caregiving families, although definitions and delivery of respite vary widely across programs and across states. In this study, all 50 states and the District of Columbia reported offering some in-home respite to caregivers under the NFCSP. States also offered other respite options, including adult day services (96%), overnight respite in a facility (84%), weekend respite or camps (69%), or other respite care (8%). Although most programs aim to offer families a choice of respite options, the choice may be limited or vary regionally depending on policy and funding decisions, and service availability in a given community. The majority of the state NFCSPs (82%) reported that caregivers were not required to live with the care receiver in order to be eligible for respite, enabling adult children or other relatives to qualify for respite assistance even if they live in separate households.

We asked state NFCSP administrators to describe the best way for a caregiver to access their program either for information or for services. Given the aging network's role in administering the NFCSP, it is not surprising that more than two-thirds cited the local AAA (69%) as the best way to access the NFCSP. Other mentioned access points included the state's toll-free telephone number (55%), other local administrative agency (27%), the Web (25%), other state agencies (20%), or other methods (14%).

TABLE 1. Caregiver Support Services Provided by State NFCSPs

Services	Program Responses*	
	n	%**
Respite Care	51	100%
Information & Assistance	50	98%
Education & Training	48	94%
Support Groups	46	90%
Care Management/Family Consultations	43	84%
Counseling (individual and/or family)	41	80%
Home Modifications	40	78%
Homemaker/Chore/Personal Care	39	77%
Assistive Technology/Emergency Response	39	77%
Transportation	35	69%
Consumable Supplies	34	67%
Legal/Financial Consultations	31	61%
Family Meetings	22	43%
Other Services	14	28%
Cash Grant	12	24%
eHealth Applications (excluding read-only websites)	6	12%

Note. Table is based on the State of the States in Family Caregiver Support Survey (Part 1, Question 18), National Center on Caregiving Caregiving, Family Caregiver Alliance, San Francisco, CA, 2004.
*N = 51. **Percentages are based on total number of responses.

We asked state NFCSP program administrators whether or not all family caregivers eligible for the program have access to the same package of services. The great majority of respondents (39 states; 78%) reported that eligible family caregivers did not have access to the same package of services throughout their states. Only 11 states and the District of Columbia reported a consistent service package for family caregivers. As well, fewer than half of the states (21; 42%) reported that all of their states' AAAs offered each of the five specified service components within their geographic area. Of those, only six states reported that all caregivers eligible for the NFCSP had access to the same package of services.

Consumer Direction

The practice of "consumer direction" has emerged as a policy trend in HCBS programs. Consumer direction is not a single method; rather, it is a philosophical approach to paying for services or supports that shifts the locus of decision making and control from service providers and payers to consumers and families (Benjamin, 2001; Doty, 2004). The NFCSP neither precludes nor mandates consumer direction. Under the NFCSP, states have the flexibility to allow direct payments to family caregivers or to provide either a voucher or budget for goods and services (e.g., grab bars, respite care), which gives families maximum control as to how, when and to whom respite is to be provided, or the option of directly purchasing goods or services to meet their needs and those of the care receiver. States may also let individual AAAs (the local administering agency) set policy for these consumer-directed approaches. In states that enable consumers to direct their own services, the freedom to hire a family member, friend, or neighbor is viewed as a meaningful feature of choice and control (Feinberg & Newman, 2004).

Most (44 out of 51; 86%) respondents reported one or more consumer-directed options for family caregivers in their states under the NFCSP. At the time of this survey, only seven state NFCSPs had no consumer-directed options for family caregivers. Most commonly, the state NFCSPs give the family a choice of respite providers (e.g., between contract agencies such as home care agencies or independent providers) (34 states; 67%); offer a voucher or budget for respite care and supplemental services (e.g., consumable supplies, assistive devices, yard maintenance) (26 states; 51%); or provide caregivers with a menu to choose those services that best fit their needs (25 states; 49%). Fewer states permit direct payments to family members to buy goods or services (15 states and the District of Columbia; 31%). One such state example is the NFCSP in Pennsylvania, which will reimburse eligible family caregivers up to $200 per month for almost any service that supports them in their caregiving roles. The Illinois Department on Aging permits local AAAs to offer vouchers (averaging $1,000 per year) to family caregivers for goods or services ranging from respite and home modifications to haircuts and lawn care. Only six states (12%) offer a respite-only voucher or budget. For instance, respite consumers in North Dakota's NFCSP can receive up to $1,900 per year to purchase respite services from a provider of their choice.

Under the NFCSP, states have the option of paying family caregivers. Over half of the respondents (30; 59%) reported that family members are permitted to be paid under the NFCSP. Of those states, respite care is the service that family members most typically can be paid to provide (28; 93%), although some states allowed payment to families to provide personal care (14; 47%) or other services (4; 13%) and, in Pennsylvania, "any service" needed by the family.

Some state NFCSPs excluded certain family members as paid caregivers, including not allowing payment to spouses (11 out of 29 states; 38%), primary caregivers (9 out of 29; 31%), parents or guardians (4 out of 29; 14%), or minor children under the age of 18 (3 out of 29; 10%). When asked if they had special requirements in order for family members to be paid to provide care, most states that permitted payment to caregivers responded that they did not (18 out of 29 states; 62%). Three of these states indicated requirements for criminal background checks; another three states had training requirements for family caregivers. None of the state agencies on aging required physician approval prior to authorizing payment to family members.

Systems Development

Program administrators were asked their opinions about the priority (high, medium, low) their states placed on 11 long-term care issues. Among the top long-term care priorities, expanding Medicaid HCBS waivers for the elderly and adults with disabilities (51%) ranked first among NFCSP respondents, followed by expanding federally-funded family caregiver support programs (49%); integrating long-term care services (46%); establishing a single point of entry for all HCBS programs, including caregiver support (43%); and implementing an *Olmstead* plan (42%). Not surprisingly, given the economic downturn in most states at the time of this survey, lowest priority was given to expanding programs or creating other financial support for caregivers at the state level. Issues most frequently identified as low priorities were: expanding state programs, including expansion of state-funded caregiver support programs (37%) or state-funded HCBS (29%); and establishing tax credits for caregiving (24%).

When asked their views about how caregiver support programs differ from other HCBS programs in their state, most frequently mentioned was the different client population. More than three-fourths of the NFCSPs (40 out of 51, 78%) stated that their programs differ from other HCBS programs because of the explicit focus on the family or informal caregiver. Ten of the 51 NFCSPs also cited the flexibility given to states to implement the NFCSP to provide multifaceted systems of caregiver support services as a difference from other publicly-funded programs. As one NFCSP respondent noted, "*I think that this is the most important program that the aging network has done in the last 20 years in terms of crossing boundaries and starting to think of older people in terms of their families and those who support them. We are moving towards supporting families . . . and recognizing that older people are part of larger family systems. If we are successful . . . it will change the way that we deliver social services. This is working to break down some of the silos that we talk about. We are becoming more responsive as a result of supporting caregivers."*

State administrators were asked to identify the three most important organizational, programmatic, geographic, or political barriers (other than funding) that limit or prevent coordination of the NFCSP with other HCBS programs in their states from a closed list of 11 items. As shown in Table 2, the top three barriers identified were different eligibility requirements, complexity and fragmentation of services, and a different client population than in other programs. Relatively few respondents identified state regulatory or statutory requirements or the low priority given to caregiver support services as a top barrier to coordination of the NFCSP with other HCBS programs.

When NFCSP respondents were asked their opinions about the major unmet needs of family caregivers in their states, three major themes emerged. Half (26; 50%) of the states and the District of Columbia identified limited respite care options as the major unmet need. Fourteen states cited the lack of resources to provide a range of caregiver services beyond just respite care, such as programs for working caregivers or providing culturally appropriate services. Thirteen state NFCSP respondents also believed that the lack of public awareness about caregiver issues and programs was the major unmet need of families.

In the telephone follow-up interviews, respondents were asked to identify the three main challenges to implementing family caregiver support services in their states. Four main themes emerged, consistent with state respondents' views on unmet caregiver needs. The majority of respondents (28 out of 51; 55%) reported inadequate funding. Lack of information and outreach to the public was viewed as a top challenge by nearly half of the NFCSP respondents (24 out of 51; 47%). Program administrators consistently commented that many families who might benefit from their programs and services did not know where to go for help. Nearly one-third (16 out of 51; 31%) of the states and the District of Columbia expressed the difficulty of providing services when many caregivers don't identify with the term "family caregiver." Rather, family members view themselves as the husband, wife, or daughter and may not recognize their own support needs or that programs could assist them in the care of their relatives. One-fourth (13 out of 51; 26%) of the

TABLE 2. Barriers That Limit/Prevent Coordination of the NFCSP with Other States' HCBS Programs*

Barrier	Program Responses**	
	n	%***
Different eligibility requirements	27	53%
Complexity and fragmentation of services	23	45%
Different client population than in other programs	23	45%
Different reporting requirements/capabilities	18	35%
Organizational cultural differences	13	26%
Staff have too many responsibilities	10	20%
Lack of access to adequate computer technology and support	7	14%
Federal regulatory or statutory requirements	6	12%
Lack of knowledge of opportunities for coordination	6	12%
State regulatory or statutory requirements	5	10%
Other	4	8%
Low priority given to caregiver support services	2	4%

Note: Table is based on the State of the States in Family Caregiver Support Survey (Part 1, Question 26), National Center on Caregiving, Family Caregiver Alliance, San Francisco, CA, 2004. *Excludes funding. **$N = 51$. ***Percentages are based on total number of responses.

states and the District of Columbia noted that providing explicit support for family and friends of frail elders represented a paradigm shift; these state administrators found the notion of serving this new client population of caregivers to be a main challenge.

CONCLUSIONS

This study profiled the experiences of all 50 states and the District of Columbia in providing services to a new client population: the family or informal caregiver of older people. All states now provide some explicit caregiver support services as a result of the passage of the NFCSP in 2000. However, in this 50-state study and in previous case study research (Feinberg & Newman, 2004), state program administrators identified the tension between serving the older person, the traditional client, and explicitly addressing the family caregiver's needs as distinct from, but related to, the needs of the older person, which is the new mandate under the NFCSP.

The NFCSP was found to stimulate service development, and to expand the range and scope of services and service options to caregivers in states where informal caregiver support services existed before the establishment of the NFCSP. To make the most use of the limited new funding, some states made the policy choice to coordinate their NFCSP with other publicly funded programs that either explicitly target support services to family caregivers, or include respite and other supports as components of larger HCBS programs. In other states, the NFCSP now provides services not available previously. Because the federal funds are targeted to those in greatest need, intended to leverage other resources and focused on core caregiver services, the NFCSP has the potential to be a vital resource for caregiving families of older persons.

This study further shows that while there is increasing availability of caregiver support services as a result of the NFCSP, there is also a great unevenness in services and service options for family caregivers across the states and within states. As well, while the NFCSP has fostered the utilization of consumer direction in caregiving programs, states differed in the extent to which they offer these options to family members. Prior research in 10 states (Feinberg & Newman, 2004) found that during the start-up phase of the NFCSP, states faced the challenge of whether to give AAAs maximum flexibility to develop individualized approaches to meet caregiver needs or setting statewide standards and uniformity so that family caregivers could access a core set of support services and service delivery options regardless of where in the state they lived. In this 50-state study, the thrust continued toward local flexibility in service design, resulting in an inconsistent range of services and service options varying by locality.

The modest level of NFCSP funding was found to leave gaps in caregiver services that vary substantially from state to state as well as within states. As a result, the inadequate resource base of the NFCSP greatly constrains the potential impact of the program. In the majority of states, caregivers in different parts of the state could not access the same package of support services under the new NFCSP. At a practical level, such service gaps and variations pose challenges for families by limiting choices for needed supports. Service inequities may also place more pressure on already strained families and compromise the ability to care for a loved one.

To effect broad policy reform and systems change, such that family caregivers are seen as true partners in long-term care, the funding level of the NFCSP will need to be raised. Ensuring that families who need help have access to at least a core minimum of service options, regardless of where they live, is a necessary first step in responding to the multifaceted needs of family caregivers. Further, increasing funds for the NFCSP can help to sustain families in their caregiving roles, in turn reducing the fiscal pressures on Medicaid and other state-funded HCBS programs at both the federal and state levels. Currently, because of limited NFCSP funding, many states rely on these other federal and state-funded HCBS programs that generally do not provide explicit support to caregiving families, other than respite benefits (Whittier, Scharlach, & Dal Santo, 2005). Congress has taken initial steps to recognize that additional funds for the NFCSP are necessary. For example, the Ronald Reagan Alzheimer's Breakthrough Act, bipartisan legislation introduced in both the 108th Congress (S.2533/H.R.4595) and the 109th Congress (S.602/H.R.1262), would double the NFCSP's initial authorization to $250 million. This increase is essential for the program to begin to achieve its aims and make measurable differences in the lives of family caregivers of frail elders.

Outreach to informal caregivers specifically, and to the public in general, is crucial to ensuring that families and friends access information and services early in the caregiving process, and have the supports they need to sustain them adequately in the caregiving role. In this study, lack of public awareness about the NFCSP and caregiving issues, including the notion that caregivers don't self-identify with the term "caregiver," was a recurring theme: as a major unmet need of caregivers, and as a challenge to implementing the NFCSP in the states.

Despite the mandate to develop a multifaceted system of explicit support services for caregivers, less than half the state NFCSPs were found to utilize a uniform assessment tool to assess caregiver needs. Establishing a national framework for caregiver assessment, based on a clinically-relevant and outcome-driven knowledge management system, would be a worthwhile investment for the NFCSP to target service interventions and to develop better and more consistent data to support and drive decision making. Ultimately, consistent approaches to caregiver assessment in all HCBS programs will enable family caregivers to obtain needed support, strengthen their ability to ensure optimal outcomes and quality of care for the care receiver, remain in the caregiving role as along as appropriate, and provide solid information to policymakers and program administrators intent on improving the effectiveness of HCBS.

Our current HCBS system relies heavily on family and informal caregivers. In the future, informal caregivers will remain the most important source of assistance for older people who need long-term care, and caregivers' own needs for direct help and support will likely intensify as they attempt to balance competing demands of work, family, and other responsibilities. Without adequate recognition of the legitimate support needs of family and informal caregivers and additional investments in services and strategies (e.g., tax and other financial incentives, family-leave policies), the reforms underway in HCBS may not be as effective and meaningful to American families. Increasing funds for the NFCSP could serve to promote systems change and a family-centered approach to HCBS by recognizing the interconnectedness of the consumer and his or her informal care network. In turn, such investments could prevent much higher Medicaid and HCBS expenditures that might be necessitated if informal caregivers became sick themselves or unavailable (Vladeck, 2004). If we are serious about reducing fragmentation in home and community-based care and recognizing the legitimate needs of informal caregivers, then assessment of caregiver needs and explicit caregiver support services should be integrated into HCBS. A family-centered approach to HCBS should be considered as states continue to pursue the goal of reforming the long-term care system. That is what most American families value and want.

AUTHOR NOTES

Lynn Friss Feinberg, MSW, is Deputy Director, National Center on Caregiving, Family Caregiver Alliance. She can be contacted at Family Caregiver Alliance, 180 Montgomery Street, Suite 1100, San Francisco, CA 94104 (E-mail: lfeinberg@caregiver.org).

Sandra Newman, MPH, is a former Policy Specialist at the National Center on Caregiving. She now is Director of Medical Practice Affairs, California Academy of Family Physicians, 1520 Pacific Avenue, San Francisco, CA 94109 (E-mail: snewman@familydocs.org).

Funding for this project was provided in part by a grant, number 90-CG-2631, from the Administration on Aging, Department of Health and Human Services. The views expressed are those of the authors and do not necessarily reflect the views of the Administration. The authors thank Leslie Gray and Karen Kolb for their invaluable assistance with this study.

REFERENCES

Aneshensel, C. S., Pearlin, L. I., Mullan, J. T., Zarit, S. H., & Whitlatch, C .J. (1995). *Profiles in caregiving: The unexpected career.* San Diego: Academic Press.

Benjamin, A. E. (2001). Consumer-directed services at home: A new model for persons with disabilities. *Health Affairs, 20*: 80-85.

Doty, P. (2004). *Consumer-directed home care: Effects on family caregivers.* San Francisco: Family Caregiver Alliance.

Feinberg, L. F., & Newman, S. L. (2004). A study of 10 states since passage of the National Family Caregiver Support Program: Policies, perceptions, and program development. *The Gerontologist, 44*: 760-769.

Feinberg, L. F., Newman, S. L., Gray, L., Kolb, K. N., & Fox-Grage, W. (2004). *The state of the states in family caregiver support: A 50-state study.* San Francisco: Family Caregiver Alliance.

Glaser, B., & Strauss, A. (1967). *Discovery of Grounded Theory.* Chicago: Aldine.

Levine, C. (2004). The loneliness of the long-term caregiver. In C. Levine (Ed.), *Always on call: When illness turns families into caregivers* (pp. 99-107). Nashville, TN: Vanderbilt University Press.

Schultz, R., Newsom, J. T., Mittlemark, M., Burton, L. C., Hirsch, C. H., & Jackson, S. (1997). Health effects of caregiving: The caregiver health effects study. *Annals of Behavioral Medicine, 19*: 110-116.

Thompson, L. (2004). *Long-term care: Support for family caregivers.* Washington, DC: Georgetown University, Long-Term Care Financing Project.

U.S. Department of Health and Human Services (2002). *Delivering the promise: Self-evaluation to promote community living for people with disabilities.* Washington, DC: Author.

Vladeck, B. C. (2004). You can't get there from here: Dimensions of caregiving and dementias of policymaking. In C. Levine (Ed.), *Family caregivers on the job: Moving beyond ADLs and IADLs* (pp. 123-137). New York: United Hospital Fund.

Wakabayashi, C., & Donato, K. M. (2004). *The consequences of caregiving for economic well-being in women's later life.* Houston, TX: Rice University, Department of Sociology.

Whittier, S., Scharlach, A., & Dal Santo, T. S. (2005). Availability of caregiver support services: Implications for implementation of the National Family Caregiver Support Program. *Journal of Aging & Social Policy, 17(1)*: 45-62.

doi:10.1300/J031v18n03_07

Families, Work, and an Aging Population: Developing a Formula That Works for the Workers

Donna L. Wagner, PhD

Towson University

SUMMARY. This article examines the intersection of family caregiving, work, and long-term care. Supporting families who provide care in order to minimize negative work effects while enhancing the acceptability of care options is of common concern to employers, state and federal policymakers, and the homecare professionals in the community-based care system. The contribution of families to the long-term care system, how employer policies have developed, how the public policy agenda has addressed family caregiving, and the importance of a more effective partnership on the state level are discussed. doi:10.1300/J031v18n03_08 *[Article copies available for a fee from The Haworth Document Delivery Service: 1-800-HAWORTH. E-mail address: <docdelivery@haworthpress.com> Website: <http://www.HaworthPress.com> © 2006 by The Haworth Press, Inc. All rights reserved.]*

KEYWORDS. Working caregivers, workplace eldercare, long-term care services, aging workforce

---

[Haworth co-indexing entry note]: "Families, Work, and an Aging Population: Developing a Formula That Works for the Workers." Wagner, Donna L. Co-published simultaneously in *Journal of Aging & Social Policy* (The Haworth Press, Inc.) Vol. 18, No. 3/4, 2006, pp. 115-125; and: *Family and Aging Policy* (ed: Francis G. Caro) The Haworth Press, Inc., 2006, pp. 115-125. Single or multiple copies of this article are available for a fee from The Haworth Document Delivery Service [1-800-HAWORTH, 9:00 a.m. - 5:00 p.m. (EST). E-mail address: docdelivery@haworthpress.com].

Available online at http://jasp.haworthpress.com
© 2006 by The Haworth Press, Inc. All rights reserved.
doi:10.1300/J031v18n03_08

INTRODUCTION

This article reviews the contributions of families to the long-term care system and the importance of their efforts, employer-based initiatives to minimize the adverse affects of family care on the workplace, and national and state-level policies that have been discussed or implemented. The article concludes with suggestions for strategies and policies to support families who work at family care and within the nation's workplaces.

EMPLOYED FAMILY CAREGIVERS

Both the 1997 and 2004 National Alliance for Caregiving (NAC)/ AARP surveys of family caregivers found that the majority of caregivers were employed or had been employed at some time during the duration of their caregiving. Many of the approximately 60% of family caregivers who were employed reported that there were times when providing family care and managing their work responsibilities were incompatible and accommodations were necessary. In the 2004 survey, 57% reported that they had to go in late to work, leave work early, or take time off to provide needed care.

While estimates of the percent of the workforce involved in eldercare varies, a conservative estimate of the percentage of the workforce involved in caregiving at any given time is 13% and expected to increase in the future (Neal & Wagner, 2001).

Employed caregivers are providing a range of support services to their older family members. The contributions to the care of an older person vary little between employed and non-working family caregivers (Stoller, 1983; Matthews, Werkner, & Delaney, 1989, for example). For many employed caregivers, however, the care comes at a price. Many caregivers must make accommodations at work. In the 1997 study of caregivers conducted by the NAC and AARP, 10% of the employed caregivers reported they had taken leaves of absence or early retirement as a result of caregiving; in the 2004 survey, 17% of the respondents reported that they had been required to take a leave of absence in order to continue their caregiving duties.

The consequences of caring and working are both personal and work-related. In the personal realm, working caregivers may need to put career plans on hold as a result of family caregiving responsibilities. These caregivers are incurring costs in·terms of money and time. Many working caregivers report that they no longer have time for personal leisure or professional development activities.

When asked what would make life easier for them, working caregivers consistently report that flexible work hours are important as is the ability to take time off when required. Of increasing importance to employed caregivers is access to "decision-support services" such as help with completing insurance paperwork and managing financial matters, elder law services, and access to geriatric care management services (Wagner, 2000).

EMPLOYERS' RESPONSES TO CAREGIVING EMPLOYEES

Large employers began to design programs to address the needs of caregiving employees in the mid-1980s. The first employer-based program was started by Hallmark in 1986 and consisted of a family resource and referral center. In 1987, Herman Miller started an eldercare resource and referral program for its employees, and in 1988, IBM began an eldercare program for its workers. In a recent Society for Human Resource Management (SHRM) survey of its members, 25% reported that they had some type of eldercare program in place. The growth of workplace eldercare programs was also fueled by organized labor through collective bargaining and related to the following corporate goals: recruitment, retention, and loyalty of employees (Galinksy & Stein, 1990; Wagner, 2000).

Employers have also been instructed by estimates of the overall costs to business of caregiving employees. Scharlach, Lowe, and Schneider (1991) estimated that an employee who was providing care for a family member was costing, on average, $2,500. These costs were based on estimates of lost productivity, lost work hours, supervisory costs, etc. The 1997 MetLife Study of Employer Costs for Working Caregivers estimated that lost productivity, absenteeism, and turnover were costing the nation's employers between $11.4 billion and $29 billion annually.

The effort of employers to address the needs of their caregiving employees has primarily involved the use of vendors who provide services to the employees for a negotiated per capita fee. The most popular model, fashioned after corporate child care services, was the resource and referral model; a set of services designed to provide help and reassurance along with contact information for community services. More recently, some employers have moved to the decision support service model that provides access to geriatric care managers, elder law attorneys, or professionals to help with insurance paperwork

Although these employer-based programs have primarily been managed privately without involvement of the public sector aging network of services, referrals rely on this network of services to supply needed supports to the elder and/or caregiver. Two area agencies have been active in serving as direct vendors to employers, New York City and the Atlanta regional area agencies on aging. And, while many area agencies on aging have expressed interest in serving the needs of employees, few have been successful in negotiating contracts with employers. We are beginning to see, however, some progress as area agencies set aside funding from the National Family Caregivers Support Program to hire staff and develop programs to meet the needs of employed caregivers. Barriers to effective public-private partnerships in this area have included inadequate knowledge on the part of employers regarding the public system of aging services, cultural differences between corporations and public-sector organizations, and established relationships between corporate decision-makers and national vendors. At this time, one of the more innovative partnerships is between Fannie Mae, a large employer, and a local aging organization, Iona House. Iona House provides a full-time case manager to Fannie Mae to meet the information and service needs of their employees (communication with program director, M. Stone).

Whatever the model, these employer-based initiatives, while likely helpful for the small number of employees who use them, do little to address the growing and widespread problems associated with family care and work. Since most employees work for small or mid-sized employers, the majority of family caregivers lack access to employer-based programs. These programs, often priced on a per capita basis, may serve as little as 1% to 2% of the workforce for any given employer (Wagner, 2000). In addition, these programs have not been evaluated objectively to determine their overall effectiveness at achieving the employers' goals.

Employer efforts have also, for the most part, been separate from governmental policies designed to help families deal with external forces of social change. These policies, most notably, The Family and Medical Leave Act, have emerged in parallel with the development of workplace programs to support family caregivers. And, interestingly, the evolution of workplace programs has occurred separately and without coordination with the governmental-based policies for families that are imposed on the larger employer.

The effect of workplace eldercare on job performance, retention, and productivity indicators is unclear as is the relative importance of these programs for the users. Do users of workplace eldercare, for example, have an easier time managing the intersection of work and family? Are the models that are in place today, which were developed 20 years ago, appropriate for today's workforce? These questions have not been addressed in a systematic way, in large part because the employer response has occurred within private, propriety systems and independent from a public response to the same population.

GOVERNMENTAL POLICIES RELATED TO WORKING CAREGIVERS

The United States lacks a comprehensive long-term care system, relying, instead, on a fragmented and complicated system of limited home- and community-based service support for income-eligible elders and private-pay options for others. For family caregivers, this approach to long term-care often means out-of-pocket payments for goods and services in addition to the assistance provided with instrumental activities of daily living and personal care.

Two major federal programs have been enacted to address the needs of family caregivers: the National Family Caregiver Support Program (NFCSP) passed in 2000 and begun in 2001, and the Family and Medical Leave Act (FMLA) passed in 1993.

The National Family Caregiver Support Program

The National Family Caregiver Support Program (NFCSP) was passed by Congress in 2001 as a public recognition of the importance of family caregivers. This program mandates that each area agency on aging design and implement programs that support family caregivers, thus extending the population served by this national network of aging service organizations. Program mandates also encourage area agencies on aging to target their efforts at those with the most financial need, further limiting the utility of this program for the millions of employed family caregivers. For information about implementation of the NFCSP, see "Preliminary Experiences of the States in Implementing the National Family Caregiver Support Program: A 50-State Study" in this volume.

The Family and Medical Leave Act

The Family and Medical Leave Act (FMLA), passed in 1993, provides job protection for workers who must take leaves of absence for up to 12 weeks from their work as a result of personal or family illness. This federal law does not include provisions for payment while on leave and applies only to employers with more than 50 employees. To put the U.S. FMLA in perspective, 139 countries provide paid leave for illness (Heymann et al., 2005). The United States does not require paid leave for short or long-term illness and only provides, through the FMLA, job protection for those workers who work for employers with more than 50 workers. And, ". . . . . Of the three industrialized nations in the world without paid leave, the United States is the richest and strongest of all" (Wisensale, 2001).

Of the 35 million workers who have used the FMLA since it began in 1993, only 6% used the FMLA to care for an ill spouse and 13% to care for an ill parent (Casta, 2000). Unpaid leave is an expensive luxury for many family caregivers.

There are other family leave issues that require attention as well. The current definition of "family" is not relevant for many American workers. As our families undergo demographic and structural changes, the definition of family needs expanding, and leave policies need to keep pace with this expansion. Step-parents and siblings, unmarried life partners, and other relationships within the "new" American family need to be seen as legitimate family care situations. And, in an aging society, it is likely that some older people will be supported not by family members, but by fictive kin. Currently, an estimated 5%-10% of older adults in the community receive ongoing support from a friend or neighbor (Barker, 2002). For more information on the Family and Medical Leave Act, see "What Role for the Family and Medical Act in Long-Term Care Policy?" in this volume.

State Government Initiatives

Connecticut was the first state to pass a family and medical leave provision for state employees in 1987. By 1999, 19 states had passed state family and medical leave provisions more generous than the FMLA. In 2004, the State of California began a paid family leave program, the first in the nation that provides a portion of wages for up to six weeks of leave per year. The paid leave program in California is completely paid for by the workers who are assessed an average of $27 per year for participation. Administered through the State Disability Insurance program, almost all workers are covered and may use the provisions to care for an ill child, parent, spouse, or domestic partner. The program pays up to 55% of the wage or salary of the worker for up to six weeks.

There are 40 states with laws that allow public employees to use their own sick leave to care for sick relatives and three states that require private employers to allow employees to use their own paid sick leave for family care (Bell & Newman, 2003). This means that a large number of employees in the United States are faced with the equally onerous choice of either taking unpaid leave or lying about their absence when family members need care. States have begun statewide respite programs and initiatives better to support family caregivers, and some have begun to explore paid leave options fashioned after the California experiment.

State policies may offer the most promise for the working caregivers and the long-term care system. The National Governors' Association (NGA) has recognized the importance of addressing the issues of caregiving and has developed a set of recommendations for both the family caregiver and the professional caregiver (NGA, 2004), recognizing that state governments have an important stake in the long-term care system. Through Medicaid waivers and state funds, state policymakers have developed a mix of home- and community-based services for persons with long-term care needs and have taken on an expanded role in innovative long-term care options (Smith et al., 2000).

In an issue brief prepared about state policies, the NGA suggests a number of programs and initiatives that can be undertaken by state policymakers and identifies innovative programs currently in place at the state level. For example, respite care is an important support for family caregivers. In 44 states, respite services are included in the Medicaid waiver programs, and in some states, a lifespan respite approach is used to coordinate the various funding available to respite care and ensure its availability for all ages of care recipients. In addition to expanded family and medical leave policies for unpaid and paid medical leave, state policymakers are encouraged to use state revenue funds to support family caregivers and to provide tax credits or tax deductions for caregiving expenses. And finally, policymakers are encouraged to use public/private partnerships and public awareness programs to enhance the support available to family caregivers (NGA, 2004).

POLICY OPTIONS FOR THE FUTURE

Interests shared by state policymakers and corporate decision-makers include the following:

- Keeping as many people working in the local economy as possible in order to foster and maintain a stable economy;
- Keeping total health costs low in order to sustain good health among the working population and their family dependents;
- Designing a cost-effective strategy for long-term care services that meets the needs of consumers without undue burden on the families, the tax payer, or the employer; and
- Maintaining a skilled, seasoned, and productive workforce over time.

Family policy that moves a state ahead in each of these goals is a critical element in sustained economic development over time.

Some states are farther along at recognizing the link between family policy and a sound economy than others. The NGA Aging Initiative with its focus on strategies that can be used by governors to support the family caregiver and address the shortages and problems associated with paid homecare workers is a good starting point to a discussion that needs to take place between policymakers and corporate decision-makers. The broad focus put forth by the NGA on improving community care, supporting family and paid care workers, health promotion, and personal financial planning provides a framework for discussion and flexibility for each state to design its own response.

In developing a statewide coalition of interest and action, the following key elements of a coalition, including large employers and state policymakers, should pursue the following:

- Linkages to home- and community-based services through the work place;
- Affordable and accessible homecare options;
- Access to caregiver support programs for employees of small and mid-sized employers; and
- Wage replacement and paid health care benefit options for workers who take leaves from their jobs to care.

Working together, the states and the business community could reduce the duplication of efforts that are present when employers invest in their own linkage system to home- and community-based services, and through joint efforts, help to support those employees who do not work for companies with work-family programs or benefits. The partnership could also foster more strategic investment in long-term care on both the private and public levels in a way that sustains the workforce in the long term and reduces the burden on the family.

States could also provide leadership in the development and support of research needed to examine the best practices for employed caregivers–research that has to date been absent. The data collected about intervention models in the workplace are largely consumer satisfaction based indicators with no objective outcome measures that relate to work place productivity, retention, or other outcomes of importance to the employer, or any outcome data that examines, over time, the mitigation of negative family or personal effects of the users. States could foster these important inquiries through partnerships with the business community to ensure that the investments in these services have a return on investment that merits their continuation or to explore other ways to maximize both the public and private investment in family care participation in the long-term care system.

CONCLUSION

The federal policies for family caregivers have been lagging behind the state policy development. The National Family Caregiving Support Program designated family caregivers as a "legitimate" service group for area agencies on aging and allocated funds to these agencies to support family caregivers. It is likely that few family caregivers understand or know that they are benefiting from this new legislation, but most family caregivers are aware of the job protection provided by the federal Family and Medical Leave Act. Unfortunately, for many family caregivers, taking unpaid leave is not possible.

Large employers, concerned about the productivity of their workforces, their ability to recruit and retain workers, and the future issues associated with an aging workforce have begun work-family programs and help family caregivers get the support they need in the community. This parallel private system relies, in part, on an under-funded public system inadequate to meet the growing needs of elders or their caregivers.

By including the family caregiving issues of workers in economic development planning, we can move the discussion and range of options from their current "service-oriented" base to a more prominent area of policy related to the continued productivity of the workforce and overall economic stability (Wagner, 2001). Family caregivers, employers, and state long-term care policymakers have been working independently of one another to address problems common to each. The intersecting issues of paid work, family care, and long-term care are of central importance to the government, employers, and American families. Designing policies that will ensure a stable economy, strong families, and an effective long-term care system is a job that requires the coordinated efforts of all stakeholders involved.

AUTHOR NOTE

Donna L. Wagner, PhD, is Professor of Gerontology and Director of Gerontology at Towson University in Maryland. She can be reached at Towson University, 8000 York Road, Towson, MD 21252-0001 or by e-mail at dwagner@towson.edu.

REFERENCES

Barker, J. C. (2002). Neighbors, friends, and other nonkin caregivers of community-living dependent elders. *Journal of Gerontology: Social Sciences, 57B (3)*: S158-S167.

Bell, L. & Newman, S. (2003). *Paid family and medical leave: Why we need it, how we can get it.* San Francisco, CA: Family Caregiver Alliance.

Casta, N. (2000). *Highlights of the 2000 U.S. Department of Labor Report: Balancing the needs of families and employers: Family and medical leave surveys.* National Partnership for Women and Families. Retrieved April, 20, 2005: www.nationalpartnership.org.

Galinsky, E., & Stein, P. J. (1990). The impact of human resource policies on employees: Balancing work/family life. *Journal of Family Issues, 11*: 368-383.

Heymann, J., Earle, A, Simmons, S, Breslow, S, & Kuehnhoff, A. (2005). *The work, family and equity index: Where does the United States stand globally?* Boston, MA: The Project on Global Working Families, Harvard School of Public Health.

Matthews, S.H., Werkner, J.E., & Delaney, P.J. (1989). Relative contributions of help by employed and nonemployed sisters to their elderly parents. *Journal of Gerontology: Social Sciences, 44*, S36-S44.

MetLife, Inc. (1997). *The MetLife study of employer costs for working caregivers.* Westport, CT: Author.

MetLife, Inc. (2004). *Miles Away: The MetLife study of long distance caregivers.* Westport, CT: Author.

National Alliance for Caregiving/AARP. (1997) *Family caregiving in the U.S: Findings from a national study.* Bethesda, MD: Author.

National Alliance for Caregiving/AARP. (2004). *Caregiving in the U.S.* Bethesda, MD: Author.

National Governors Association (NGA) (2004). *State support for family caregivers and paid home-care workers: Issue Brief.* www.nga.org.

Neal, M. B., & Wagner, D. L. (2001). *Working Caregivers: Issues, Challenges, and Opportunities for the Aging Network.* Issue Brief, National Family Caregiver Support Program, Administration on Aging, Washington, DC: www.aoa.gov.

Scharlach, A. E., Lowe, B. F., & Schneider, E. L. (1991). *Elder care and the workforce: Blueprint for action.* Lexington, MA: Lexington.

Select Committee on Aging. (1987). *Exploding the Myths: Caregiving in America.* Committee Publication No. 99-611. Washington, DC: Government Printing Office.

Smith, G., O'Keefe, J., Carpenter, L, Doty, P., & Kennedy, G. (2000). *Understanding Medicaid home and community services: A primer.* Washington, DC: Department of Health and Human Services (ASPE).

Stoller, E.P. (1983). Parental caregiving by adult children. *Journal of Marriage and the Family,* 45: 851-858.

Wagner, D. L., & Hunt, G. G. (1994). The use of workplace eldercare programs by employed caregivers. *Research on Aging, 16:* 69-84.

Wagner, D. L. (2000). The development and future of workplace eldercare. In *Dimensions of family caregiving: A look into the future.* Westport, CT: MetLife Mature Market Institute.

Wagner, D. L. (2001). *Enhancing state initiatives for working caregivers.* Issue Brief. Family Caregiver Alliance, San Francisco, CA: www.caregiver.org.

Wagner, D.L. (2004). The financial impact of caregiving. In *Always on call: When illness turns families into caregivers,* C. Levine (Ed.). Nashville, TN: Vanderbilt Univ. Press.

Wisensale, S. K. (2001). *Family leave policy: The political economy of work and family in America.* Armonk, NY: M.E. Sharpe, Inc.

doi:10.1300/J031v18n03_08

Family and Friends as Respite Providers

Carol J. Whitlatch, PhD

Margaret Blenkner Research Institute, Benjamin Rose

Lynn Friss Feinberg, MSW

National Center on Caregiving, Family Caregiver Alliance

SUMMARY. Consumer-directed service options in home- and community-based care are increasingly available to adults with chronic conditions and cognitive impairments and to their family caregivers. Few studies, however, examine the experience of family caregivers who, when given a choice of providers of respite assistance (i.e., relief from the stress of providing constant care), prefer to hire family or friends rather than service providers. This study describes the in-home respite experience of family caregivers served by California's Caregiver Resource Centers "direct-pay" program who hire family or friends (n = 39) or service providers (n = 77) to provide in-home respite assistance. Findings revealed similarities between the two groups with few exceptions: caregivers who hired family or friends reported poorer physical health, were slightly more satisfied with the respite assistance, and received more hours of respite at a lower unit cost. These findings lend support to consumer-directed respite service options where family caregivers are given flexible alternatives that may act to remove barriers to respite service availability and use. doi:10.1300/J031v18n03_09 *[Article copies available for a fee from The Haworth Document Delivery Service: 1-800-HAWORTH. E-mail address: <docdelivery@haworthpress.com> Website: <http://www.HaworthPress.com> © 2006 by The Haworth Press, Inc. All rights reserved.]*

[Haworth co-indexing entry note]: "Family and Friends as Respite Providers." Whitlatch, Carol J., and Lynn Friss Feinberg. Co-published simultaneously in *Journal of Aging & Social Policy* (The Haworth Press, Inc.) Vol. 18, No. 3/4, 2006, pp. 127-139; and: *Family and Aging Policy* (ed: Francis G. Caro) The Haworth Press, Inc., 2006, pp. 127-139. Single or multiple copies of this article are available for a fee from The Haworth Document Delivery Service [1-800-HAWORTH, 9:00 a.m. - 5:00 p.m. (EST). E-mail address: docdelivery@haworthpress.com].

KEYWORDS. Respite care, home-based care, community-based care, family caregivers, service providers

INTRODUCTION

It is well-documented that caring for a relative with cognitive impairment can lead to compromised mental and physical health due to the impaired adult's behavioral and personality changes, constant and long-term care demands, and the high costs of care (Aneshensel et al., 1995; Schulz et al., 1995). Family caregivers often identify respite assistance as one of their most pressing needs so that they might have a break from the stress of constant care (Lawton et al., 1989). (For purposes of this study, "respite" is defined as "substitute care or supervision in support of the caregiver for the purposes of providing relief from the stresses of constant care provision and so as to enable the caregiver to pursue a normal routine and responsibilities." Chapter 1658, Statutes of 1984, as amended by Chapter 775, Statutes of 1988 and Chapter 7, California Welfare & Institutions code, Section 4362 et al., 1992.) The variety and flexibility of respite services contribute to its value for families whose situations differ dramatically from one another and over time (Feinberg & Kelly, 1995). Yet, the effectiveness of respite for reducing caregiving's physical and emotional effects is not clearly substantiated (Lawton et al., 1989), possibly due to the reluctance, underutilization, delayed and/or inappropriate use of respite services by families (Gwyther, 1994).

One option for improving accessibility and utilization of respite assistance is to provide greater access to and choice about various in-home respite options. It has been suggested that when given a choice between agency-based respite and the independent provider or "direct-pay" model (where families hire and supervise their own aides), most families prefer the latter mode because they retain control, choice, potential for individualization, flexibility, and more consistency of providers (Doty et al., 1996; Gwyther, 1994), including the option to hire family and friends. Given the mutual preference of caregivers and care recipients for family members to provide care, it makes sense that a preferred option for many caregivers would be to have family and/or friends provide hands-on care for their relatives that would allow them to have some time away (i.e., respite) from their on-going care situation (Dale et al., 2003; Feinberg & Whitlatch, 2002).

Few studies focus on care options that allow family caregivers to hire family and/or friends as respite workers. More common are programs and studies that examine outcomes from the perspective of persons with disabilities who have access to consumer-directed options. Family caregiver outcomes are rarely studied within these consumer-directed programs. One exception is the work of Foster et al. (2005), which examined family caregiver outcomes within the Cash and Counseling (C&C) model where the Medicaid beneficiary receives a monthly allowance to hire personal assistance service workers (including relatives) and to purchase assistive devices, care supplies, or home modifications. Results suggest that family caregivers are indirectly and positively affected by their relative's access to and use of consumer-directed options; thus, family caregiver outcomes are better when C&C beneficiaries direct their own personal care services. Unfortunately, little is known about outcomes for family caregivers who have choice and flexibility in making decisions about service preferences and respite needs.

Data for the present study are taken from an investigation of the in-home respite experience of non-Medicaid eligible middle-income family caregivers served by California's model system of 11 Caregiver Resource Centers (see Feinberg & Kelly, 1995 for a full description of the CRC respite program). The purpose of the study was to compare the in-home respite experiences of caregivers using the CRC direct-pay mode with caregivers using the agency-based option (Feinberg & Whitlatch, 1998). Specifically, the vendor (i.e., agency-based) in-home respite program provides caregivers with vouchers to purchase service hours from homecare agencies under subcontract with a CRC. In the "direct-pay" (i.e., consumer-directed or independent provider) program, caregivers are given vouchers to hire and manage their own respite workers, including payments to family members or friends to provide respite care. Findings indicated that caregivers preferred the consumer-directed mode (i.e., direct-pay), which was found to provide more hours of respite at a significantly lower unit cost per hour of service. Additionally, we wondered about the many direct-pay caregivers who knew their in-home aides previously, and if there were differences between caregivers who hired family and friends versus those who hired service providers; were caregivers who hired family and friends "better off" in terms of well-being, finances, etc., than caregivers who hired service providers? Thus, we compare the background characteristics, levels of distress, depression, satisfaction with care, and differences in the cost and amount of respite received by family caregivers who hire family and friends versus those who hire service providers.

METHODS

Data Collection and Measures

The sample was recruited from the respite caseload of nine of the 11 California CRCs that offered both agency-based and direct-pay in-home respite assistance. California's model system of CRCs is a nationally recognized statewide program known for its development of innovative approaches to the delivery of services to support families and caregivers of adults with cognitive impairments and other chronic conditions. In the CRC system, the family caregiver is considered the client. Although CRCs provide a broad range of support services (e.g., legal consultations, counseling) and respite options (e.g., in-home, adult day, weekend), in-home respite is usually a caregiver's first choice when considering respite options.

Questionnaires were mailed to all 216 eligible respondents within the CRC system. To be eligible, family caregivers had to be: (1) the person primarily responsible for the day-to-day care of a cognitively impaired adult living in the community, and (2) receiving in-home respite from a CRC during the one-month study period. Completed data were obtained from 168 respondents. Similar to the previous findings within the CRC system (Feinberg & Kelly, 1995), more than twice as many caregivers were receiving respite from the direct-pay respite program (n = 116; 68%) than from the agency-based program (n = 52, 32%). The present study compares the experiences of caregivers from the direct-pay program who hired family or friends (n = 39; 34%) and those who hired respite aides from a homecare or other agency (n = 77; 66%).

Measures of care receiver characteristics included age, gender, diagnosis, ethnicity, and the Memory and Behavioral Problems Checklist (Zarit et al., 1980), which assesses the extent to which 25 behaviors (1 = Yes; 0 = No) characterize the care receiver during the previous week: Personal Activities of Daily Living (α = .74), Instrumental ADLs (α = .73), Cognition (α = . 78), and Problem Behaviors (α = .79).

Caregiver demographics included age, gender, relationship to the care receiver (e.g., wife, daughter, etc.), ethnicity, marital status, educational level, employment status, household income, length of time providing care, and length of time receiving CRC respite.

Caregiver respite preferences and involvement were examined using: (1) a 12-item checklist identifying the major reasons that caregivers chose the type of in-home respite care they received (e.g., safety of loved one, fit the household, etc.); (2) a single-item question identifying the "single most important reason" for choosing the type of respite they received, again using the 12-item checklist; and (3) questions adapted from the Commonwealth Fund's homecare study (1991) examining the caregiver's level of involvement in supervising his or her aide (e.g., hiring, firing, etc.).

Caregiver satisfaction was measured by asking caregivers if they were very satisfied, satisfied, or unsatisfied with 11 aspects of their respite care (e.g., number of hours, quality, etc.).

Level of caregiver distress and depression was assessed by asking caregivers about the distress they felt when they first began receiving CRC respite assistance and their current level of distress (very distressed, somewhat distressed, not very distressed, or not at all distressed). The 20-item Center for Epidemiological Studies Depression Scale (CES-D; $\alpha = .93$; Radloff, 1977) was used to measure caregiver depression including mood, feelings of guilt, worthlessness, hopelessness, loss of energy, etc. The CES-D measures current state and has been used in numerous caregiving studies (Schulz et al., 1995). Scores of 16 or higher indicate significant depressive symptoms (Radloff & Teri, 1986).

Caregiver respite service use and cost data were obtained from the existing CRC services automation system used to track CRC service usage and expenditures. Items were drawn from the database for the month caregivers completed their surveys: type of respite used (only in-home respite users were included), type of provider (direct-pay versus agency-based), hours of CRC respite used during the study period month, and hourly cost of respite care paid for by the CRC (including costs of benefits and overhead for agency-based respite).

RESULTS

1. What are the characteristics of direct-pay in-home respite users who hire family and friends (n = 39) versus those who hire service providers (n = 72)?

As shown in Table 1, caregivers who hired family and friends were very similar in their demographic characteristics to caregivers who

TABLE 1. Caregiver and Care Recipient Characteristics

Caregiver	Hired family or friends (n = 39)	Hired service providers (n = 77)
% female	76.9	72.7
% homemaker	20.5	15.8
% employed full time	10.5	22.1
Mean age (s.d.; range in years)	57.9 (13.8; 28-96)	59.5 (13.6; 22-86)
% spouse	79.5	79.2
% living with care recipient	95.0	95.0
% married	89.7	90.5
% Caucasian	73.7	72.0
Median education	"some college"	"some college"
Median annual income range	$16-20,000	$25-30,000
Mean years providing care (s.d.; range in years)	10.5 (10.3; <1-58)	9.3 (5.3; <1-35)
Number of health symptoms	3.95	3.36
Overall physical health	2.31	2.50
CESD	20.4	18.4
Current health worse than 5 years ago[a]	1.33	1.64
Health problems getting in way of CG doing things[b]	1.79	2.10
Level of distress when first received CRC respite assistance	3.26	3.36
Current level of distress	2.74	2.82
Care Recipient		
mean age (s.d.; range in years)	64.2 (15.9; 24-94)	66.8 (11.5; 31-88)
% female	38.5	46.8
Diagnosis		
Stroke	25.6	37.7
Alzheimer's disease	28.2	18.2
Other degenerative disease/dementia	23.1	19.5
Parkinson's disease and other conditions	23.9	25.7

	Mean	Range	Mean	Range	
Problem behaviors	2.9	0-7	2.7	0-8	ns
Instrumental activities of daily living	3.6	0-4	3.6	0-4	ns
Personal activities of daily living	3.3	0-4	3.0	0-4	p = .18
Cognitive difficulties	4.8	0-8	4.4	0-8	ns

[a] p = .007   [b] t = 2.18, p = .03

hired service providers. However, caregivers who hired family and friends reported significantly worse current physical health than five years previously (1.33 vs. 1.64, $p = .007$) and health problems getting "in the way of doing things" the caregiver wanted to do (1.79 vs. 2.10; $t = 2.18$, $p = .03$).

2. What reasons do caregivers give for preferring one mode of in-home respite over the other?

Caregivers in both groups (see Table 2) reported the same most important reasons for preferring the respite option they chose: safety of loved one; wanting good, reliable, and trustworthy help; and ability to choose their own home aides. Caregivers in both groups ranked "safety of their loved one" as the "single most important reason" for choosing their preferred type of CRC in-home respite, followed by good, reliable, and trustworthy help, and choice of own homecare aides.

Next, we compared group differences in the amount of control or choice a caregiver exercised with respect to in-home respite. Building upon findings from the Commonwealth Fund's 1991 study of the importance of choice in homecare programs, we created a summary variable reflecting the caregivers' "index of choice." Caregiver responses

TABLE 2. Caregiver Respite Preferences

Preferences	Hired family or friends (n = 39)		Hired service providers (n = 77)	
	% YES	Rank [a]	% YES	Rank [a]
Safety of loved one	89.5	#1 (54.1%)	92.2	#1 (42.1%)
Good, reliable, trustworthy help	86.8	#2 (27.0%)	88.3	#2 (30.3%)
Choose own homecare aide	84.2	#3 (10.8%)	75.3	#3 (10.5%)
Fit the household	65.8		54.5	
Most service for lowest cost	47.4		57.1	
Flexibility in care arrangements	42.1		40.3	
Well trained homecare aide	31.6		42.9	
Control in decision-making	28.9		46.8	
Input in care arrangements	26.3		22.1	
Unsatisfied with previous homecare	13.2		11.7	
Did not want to arrange care myself	5.3		10.4	
Agency responsible for arrangements	2.6		10.4	

[a] Caregiver ranking of single most important reason for hiring family and friends or service

were coded (yes = 1, no = 0) to indicate the amount of choice or control a caregiver exercised in five areas. In comparing caregivers who hired family and friends versus caregivers who hired service providers (data not shown), results indicated that the groups were very similar in terms of being responsible for scheduling the aide (94.9% vs. 90.8%), signing the aide's time sheet and pay check (63.9% vs. 62.9%), making sure the aide did the job the way s/he should (92.3% vs. 96.1%), and being responsible for replacing their aide if needed (76.9% vs. 80.0%). Conversely, caregivers who hired their own family members and friends were much more likely to have known their in-home respite aides before the aides started working for the caregiver (79.5% vs. 26.3%). Caregivers who chose family and friends reported having significantly more control and choice than caregivers who chose service providers in decisions related to the day-to-day management of their in-home respite aides (mean score = 4.11 vs. 3.58; t = −2.90, $p < .01$).

3. What are the caregivers' levels of distress and depression?

No significant differences were found between caregivers who hired family and friends and those who hired service providers in current and previous levels of caregiver distress or current levels of depression (see Table 1). Mean levels of depression for both groups (20.4 vs. 18.4, respectively) were above the cut-off criteria for the CES-D indicating significant symptoms of depression. Ordinary least-squares regression analyses determined the key predictors of the caregiver's current level of distress and depression (see Table 3). Results indicated that caregivers who reported feeling more distressed at the time of the survey (R^2 = .25, $p < .000$) were more distressed before they began receiving CRC respite assistance, more depressed currently, and less satisfied with CRC respite assistance. For caregiver depression (R^2 = .24, $p < .000$), results indicated that caregivers with more symptoms of depression were currently more distressed, were not as satisfied with their current aides, and felt they had more control in managing their in-home respite care.

4. What are caregivers' levels of satisfaction with the respite they receive?

As seen in Table 4, both groups of caregivers were found to be satisfied with many aspects of their respite care. Caregivers who hired family or friends were slightly more satisfied overall than caregivers who hired service providers (mean = 2.46 vs. 2.35, $t = −1.47$, $p = .14$; score

TABLE 3. Ordinary Least Squares Regression Predicting Current Levels of Caregiver Distress and Depression

Key Predictors	Current level of caregiver distress	Current level of caregiver depression
Previous level of distress	.14	–
Current level of depression	.41	–
Satisfaction with respite assistance	−.18	NS
Perception of aide's skill level	NS	−.14
Caregiver's physical health symptoms	–	NS
Current level of distress	–	.40
Caregiver willingness to assume care	–	NS
"Index of choice"	–	.18
R^2	.25 $p < .000$	.24 $p < .000$

NS = non-significant predictor that was included in the regression analysis
– = indicates that the predictor was not included in the regression analysis

of 2 equals satisfied, and a score of 3 equals very satisfied). Over 92% of caregivers in both groups were either satisfied or very satisfied with nearly all aspects of care, including the quality of care provided by their aides, tailoring the care to meet their needs, support of CRC social worker, ease of arranging homecare, amount of paperwork involved, consistency of help, safety of their relatives, and the reliability, and trustworthiness of their aides. Results of regression analyses indicated that significant predictors of caregiver satisfaction with their respite aides ($R^2 = .20$, $p < .001$) included lower distress (B = −.18, $p < .08$), feeling that their current aides did their jobs well (B = .38, $p < .001$), and higher levels of subjective health (B = .17, $p < .05$). Non-significant key predictors included the index of choice and caregiver depression.

5. Are there differences in the cost and amount of respite received for caregivers who hired family and/or friends and those who do not?

Although no significant differences were found in the amount of respite paid for by the CRCs (approximately $250 per month), caregivers

TABLE 4. Caregiver Satisfaction with CRC In-Home Respite

Respite characteristics	Hired family or friends (n = 39)			Hired service providers (n = 77)		
	Unsatisfied	Satisfied	Very Satisfied	Unsatisfied	Satisfied	Very Satisfied
Number of hours help	28.2	48.7	23.1	32.0	57.3	10.7
Spread of hours per week	10.8	56.8	32.4	17.8	65.8	16.4
Tailoring homecare	8.1	51.4	40.5	8.1	58.1	33.8
Quality	–	35.1	64.9	1.4	45.9	52.7
Support of CRC social worker	2.9	38.2	58.8	–	37.7	62.3
Ease arranging homecare	5.7	42.9	51.4	7.0	60.6	32.4
Paperwork involved	–	58.3	41.7	4.0	61.3	34.7
Consistency of help	2.9	50.0	47.1	4.2	42.3	53.5
Safety of loved one	–	27.0	73.0	1.4	39.2	59.5
Reliability	2.9	22.9	74.3	1.4	35.1	63.5
Trustworthy	2.6	23.7	73.7	1.3	33.3	65.3
Overall satisfaction	–	12.8	87.2	2.6	17.1	80.3
Unsatisfied = 1; Satisfied = 2; Very Satisfied = 3						
Mean overall satisfaction (t = −1.47, p = .14)	2.46			2.35		

who hired family and friends received more respite assistance (41.5 versus 33.25 hours per month, or 9.65 versus 7.7 hours per week; t = −1.79, p = .08). Moreover, caregivers who hired family and friends received respite at a significantly lower unit cost ($8.48 per hour vs. $12.67 per hour in 2005 U.S. dollars [adjusted from 1996 U.S. dollars for inflation using the Consumer Price Index]; p = .11).

DISCUSSION

The results of this study indicate that family caregivers who hired family and friends as respite aides (n = 39) versus caregivers who hired service providers (n = 77) were very similar in their demographic characteristics and levels of mental health and distress with few exceptions: caregivers who hired family and friends were slightly more likely to report worse current health than five years previously, to report health problems getting in the way of "doing things," to have slightly higher levels of satisfaction with the respite assistance they received, and to have exercised more control and choice in making decisions about the day-to-day management of their in-home respite aides. Results also indicate that hiring family and friends was less costly per hour of service than hiring service providers (i.e., $8.48 per hour vs. $12.67 per hour 2005 U.S. dollars) and that these caregivers received more hours of respite assistance per week (9.1 vs. 7.7 hours per week).

Similar to our previous work (Feinberg & Whitlatch, 1998), it appears that caregivers who hire family and friends may experience both cost savings and the receipt of significantly more hours of relief from the stress of constant care. Our findings are both consistent and inconsistent with those of the Cash and Counseling Demonstration Evaluation in Arkansas. Dale and colleagues (2003) report that persons receiving Medicaid Personal Assistant Services assigned to the consumer-directed treatment group were more satisfied with their care and received more paid services than consumers in the control group (i.e., the less consumer-directed option where consumers continued to use agency services), yet the consumer-directed treatment group experienced higher short-term costs. Interestingly, higher costs in the treatment group were offset by subsequent savings in nursing home use. These studies lend support to consumer-directed service models where family caregivers and/or persons with chronic conditions are given flexible options that may act to remove barriers (e.g., few available aides, limited and inflexible scheduling) to their using in-home respite and/or personal assistance services.

There is controversy surrounding the utility and acceptability of paying family and/or friends to provide respite or other homecare. Critics of paying family caregivers are concerned about appropriate public-private responsibility, increased expenditures of public dollars for services primarily provided for free by families, greater risk of fraud and abuse, and quality of care (Blaser, 1998; Linsk et al., 1992). Respite workers who are family and friends oftentimes do not have health care benefits, liability insurance, or career ladders available to them. Proponents, on the other hand, argue that paying family members to provide respite can be beneficial to both care recipients and family caregivers by increasing consumer choice, improving quality of care, expanding the limited worker supply, and sustaining the natural support system (Foster et al.,

2005; Kunkel et al., 2004; Simon-Rusinowitz et al., 1998). The results of this research support payment to family and friends to provide respite care as an option in the financing and delivery of home-based care to meet the needs and preferences of caregiving families.

The importance of consumer direction in respite care for family caregivers remains an important issue for long-term care policymakers. Respite options that include the hiring and managing of family and friends may be one way to provide access to respite care for persons otherwise unwilling to allow "strangers" into their home. This approach, however, is not preferred by or appropriate for all families; caregivers with few nearby family members or friends would be unlikely to prefer this mode. To meet the changing needs of family caregivers, practitioners must offer families access to a range of service delivery options, assess for the caregivers' preferences and abilities to direct the day-to-day management of in-home respite care, and give the caregivers the choice to hire family and/or friends as respite aides. As caregivers are given more access to and choice in their respite options and more control over care decisions, it is likely that respite care will be viewed by families as a more viable and acceptable form of assistance.

AUTHOR NOTES

Carol J. Whitlatch, PhD, is Assistant Director of the Margaret Blenkner Research Institute, Benjamin Rose. Dr. Whitlatch can be contacted at the Margaret Blenkner Research Institute, Benjamin Rose, 850 Euclid Avenue, Suite 1100, Cleveland, OH 44114- 3301(E-mail: cwhitlat@benrose.org).

Lynn Friss Feinberg, MSW, is Deputy Director, National Center on Caregiving, Family Caregiver Alliance, 180 Montgomery Street, Suite 1100, San Francisco, CA 94104 (E-mail: lfeinberg@caregiver.org).

This study was made possible in part by support from the State of California, Department of Health Services, under Agreement No. 95-23333.

REFERENCES

Aneshensel, C. S., Pearlin, L. I., Mullan, J. T., Zarit, S. H., & Whitlatch, C. J. (1995). *Profiles in Caregiving: The Unexpected Career.* New York: Academic.

Blaser, C. J. (1998). The case against paying family caregivers: Ethical and practical issues. *Generations, 22:* 65-69.

Commonwealth Fund Commission on Elderly Living Alone (1991). *The importance of choice in Medicaid home care programs: Maryland, Michigan, and Texas.* New York: Louis Harris and Associates.

Dale, S., Brown, R., Phillips, B., Schore, J., & Carlson, B. L. (2003). The effects of cash and counseling on personal care services and Medicaid costs in Arkansas. *Health Affairs–Web Exclusive, 19 November,* W3-566-575.

Doty, P., Kasper, J., & Litvak, S. (1996). Consumer directed models of personal care: Lessons from Medicaid. *The Milbank Quarterly, 74:* 337-409.

Feinberg, L. F., & Kelly, K. A. (1995). A well-deserved break: Respite programs offered by California's statewide system of caregiver resource centers. *The Gerontologist, 35:* 701-705.

Feinberg, L. F., & Whitlatch, C. J. (1998). Family caregivers and in-home respite options: The consumer-directed versus agency-based experience. *Journal of Gerontological Social Work, 30*(3): 9-28.

Feinberg, L. F., & Whitlatch, C. J. (2002). Decision-making for persons with cognitive impairment and their family caregivers. *American Journal of Alzheimer's Disease and Other Dementias, 17*(4): 237-244.

Foster, L., Brown, R., Phillips, B., & Carlson, B. L. (2005). Easing the burden of caregiving: The impact of consumer direction on primary informal caregivers in Arkansas. *The Gerontologist, 45*(4): 474-485.

Gwyther, L. (1994). Service delivery and utilization: Research directions and clinical implications. In E. Light, G. Niederehe, & B.D. Lebowitz (Eds.), *Stress effects on family caregivers of Alzheimer's patients: Research and interventions.* New York: Springer.

Kunkel, R., Applebaum, R. A., & Nelson, I. M. (2004). For love or money: Paying family caregivers. *Generations, 27:* 74-80.

Lawton, M. B., Brody, E. M., & Saperstein, A. R. (1989). A controlled study of respite services for caregivers of Alzheimer's patients. *The Gerontologist, 29:* 8-16.

Linsk, N. L., Keigher, S. M., Simon-Rusinowitz, L., & England, S. E. (1992). *Wages for caring: Compensating family care of the elderly.* New York: Praeger.

Radloff, L. S. (1977). The CES-D Scale: A self-report depression scale for research in the general population. *Applied Psychological Measurement, 1:* 385-401.

Radloff, L. S., & Terri, L. (1986). Use of the Center for Epidemiological Studies Depression Scale with older adults. *Clinical Gerontologist, 5:* 119-135.

Schulz, R., O'Brien, A. T., Bookwala, J., & Fleissner, K. (1995). Psychiatric and physical morbidity effects in Alzheimer's disease caregiving: Prevalence, correlates, and causes. *The Gerontologist, 35:* 771-791.

Simon-Rusinowitz, L., Mahoney, K., & Benjamin, A. E. (1998). Payments to families who provide care: An option that should be available. *Generations, 22:* 69-75.

Zarit, S. H., Reever, K. E., & Bach-Peterson, J. (1980). Relatives of the impaired elderly: Correlates of feelings and burden. *The Gerontologist, 20:* 649-655.

doi:10.1300/J031v18n03_09

The Family Caregiving Career: Implications for Community-Based Long-Term Care Practice and Policy

Joseph E. Gaugler, PhD

University of Minnesota

Pamela Teaster, PhD

University of Kentucky

SUMMARY. Informal (i.e., unpaid) long-term care for disabled older adults is often chronic, but it is only recently that research has considered the longitudinal implications of family caregiving. In particular, investigators have conceptualized caregiving as a "career," and within the caregiving career, a number of diverse trajectories and transitions can occur. Following a summary of these findings, this paper considers how longitudinal caregiving research can influence and potentially address key policy and practice concerns, especially in the delivery and support of community-based long-term care (CBLTC) services. It is suggested that with the refinement of the informal long-term care literature, existing policy and practice to support caregiving families can be similarly advanced. doi:10.1300/J031v18n03_10 *[Article copies available for a fee from The Haworth Document Delivery Service: 1-800-HAWORTH. E-mail address: <docdelivery@haworthpress.com> Website: <http://www.HaworthPress.com> © 2006 by The Haworth Press, Inc. All rights reserved.]*

[Haworth co-indexing entry note]: "The Family Caregiving Career: Implications for Community-Based Long-Term Care Practice and Policy" Gaugler, Joseph E., and Pamela Teaster. Co-published simultaneously in *Journal of Aging & Social Policy* (The Haworth Press, Inc.) Vol. 18, No. 3/4, 2006, pp. 141-154; and: *Family and Aging Policy* (ed: Francis G. Caro) The Haworth Press, Inc., 2006, pp. 141-154. Single or multiple copies of this article are available for a fee from The Haworth Document Delivery Service [1-800-HAWORTH, 9:00 a.m. - 5:00 p.m. (EST). E-mail address: docdelivery@haworthpress. com].

KEYWORDS. Informal long-term care, caregiving transitions, community-based long-term care

INTRODUCTION

Studies examining older persons with chronic diseases reveal that informal (i.e., unpaid) family care can entail "careers" that include a number of transitions such as onset and institutionalization, along with progression and change in the care provided (Pavalko & Woodbury, 2000; Montgomery & Kosloski, 2000; Pearlin & Aneshensel, 1994). The purpose of this article is to link emerging longitudinal research on informal long-term care with policy and practice recommendations designed to enhance the potential of CBLTC services to alleviate key negative caregiving outcomes. Incorporating important insights on the longitudinal ramifications of the caregiving career into the current programmatic emphasis of CBLTC can potentially help providers, policymakers, and researchers ascertain how such programs are most effectively delivered to families in need.

The Caregiving Career

As several researchers have emphasized (i.e., Montgomery & Kosloski, 2000; Pearlin, 1992; Pearlin & Aneshensel, 1994), family caregiving is far from static, but instead consists of a variety of stages around which a discernible career is organized. These stages include the onset of family care (which can be delineated by identifying when the individual first performs caregiving tasks, the self-definition of "caregiver," and the eventual provision of personal care; see Montgomery & Kosloski, 2000), relinquishing of at-home/community care responsibilities to residential long-term care, and bereavement. Montgomery and Kosloski (2000) further differentiate the stages prior to relinquishing at-home care with the following markers: seeking assistance and formal service use, considering nursing home placement, actual institutionalization, and termination of the caregiving role that occurs due to the death of the care recipient, recovery of the care recipient (a more likely occurrence in acute disorders when compared to chronic disorders such as dementia), or a decision by the caregiver to "quit." Certainly, these conceptualizations of the caregiving career do not denote systematic progression through each stage, but instead identify potential transitions that may influence the nature of informal care provision. Thus, the concept of career is particularly appropriate in any study of informal care and chronic disease; as family caregiving progresses, individuals may experience a change in status, or role expectations and responsibilities, as well as changes within status, such as increases or decreases in certain care demands due to the functional and cognitive deterioration of a loved one suffering from a chronic disorder.

LONGITUDINAL RESEARCH ON FAMILY CAREGIVING

The initial objective of this paper is to summarize the psychosocial and health effects of caregiving over time. While a comprehensive literature search was conducted, due to space considerations the following section highlights what we perceive as some of the key trends, studies, and findings in the literature. Several meta-analyses now exist of informal caregiving and its psychosocial and health implications (e.g., Vitaliano, Zhang, & Scanlan, 2003).

At-Home Caregiving

The bulk of longitudinal research on family care for disabled older adults focuses on those individuals providing informal assistance in at-home settings. Many of these studies have attempted to explore the "wear and tear" hypothesis. Based on classic physiological and psychosocial research on chronic stress (e.g., Pearlin, Lieberman, Menaghan, & Mullan, 1981), the wear and tear hypothesis suggests that the longer a caregiver remains in her/his role, the more likely negative outcomes will occur. Many of these efforts are cross-sectional in design and attempt to correlate duration of care indices (i.e., "How long have you been providing care to your relative?") with various measures of caregiver burden, depression, and other forms of psychosocial distress. When considered in comprehensive fashion with other variables such as care recipient functional and cognitive impairment, duration of care rarely appears as an independent, significant predictor of psychosocial outcomes (see review by Montgomery & Williams, 2001). Panel studies of dementia caregiving have instead found an adaptation effect, where caregivers who remain in follow-up intervals report decreases or stability in negative emotional and psychological outcomes (e.g., see Gaugler, Kane et al., 2005a). These studies have supported counter-hypotheses in the literature that emphasize the ability of families to tolerate once stressful situations, or to adapt to and successfully manage chronic caregiving demands and stressors. Those analyses that moved beyond traditional between-subjects models to consider intra-individual trajectories in caregivers' burden and depression found considerable change occurring, suggesting that key indicators such as care recipient functional dependencies (e.g., behavior problems; Gaugler, Kane et al., 2005a; Roth et al., 2001) may drive caregivers' psychosocial outcomes over time. Prospective longitudinal studies demonstrate similar, dynamic relationships between the physiological and subjective health implications of family caregiving and care recipient functional status over time (see Vitaliano et al., 2003).

Transitions in Caregiving

An emerging area of informal long-term care research has been the analysis of transitions and their effects on family caregivers. For example, several efforts have explored how the transition from non-caregiver to caregiver (or, from providing no activity of daily living assistance at one time point to providing help with at least one of these tasks in a subsequent interval) affects stress and negative mental health over time (e.g., Lawton, Moss, Hoffman, & Perkinson, 2000). In general, care recipients' functional dependencies appear to influence the onset of informal caregiving (e.g., a health crisis) and cause distress initially, followed by a sense of stabilization in emotional and psychological outcomes. Other studies have revealed that those individuals who experience less abrupt entries into their caregiving roles are more likely to delay nursing home placement as well as indicate decreases in emotional distress and depression over time (Burton et al., 2003; Gaugler, Zarit, & Pearlin, 2003). Taken together, the findings imply that how people assume care responsibilities or manage problems early in their careers has important longitudinal implications, particularly in chronic diseases such as dementia.

A number of studies have been conducted examining the influence of caregiving indicators (e.g., stress, sociodemographic context) on institutionalization. Earlier research had solely considered functional, sociodemographic, and service use indicators of older adults as potential predictors. However, a series of analyses considering caregiving and institutionalization has filled an important gap in the literature. In recent large-scale analyses of dementia caregiving and institutionalization, indicators of caregiver well-being (i.e., burden, self-rated health) were identified as potent predictors of placement along with care recipient behavior problems (Gaugler, Kane et al., 2003). While prior studies have approached institutionalization as the end of caregiving, recent research has implied the prolonged effects of stress following nursing home placement. A growing number of studies have indicated that various dimensions of emotional distress and psychological well-being remain relatively stable for dementia caregivers after institutionalization (e.g., Schulz et al., 2004). Moreover, institutionalization often introduces new challenges for the family caregiver as responsibilities change and roles shift (e.g., Yamamoto-Mitani, Aneshensel, & Levy-Storms, 2002), and negative interactions between family caregivers and institutional staff and poor perceptions of care can have powerful and negative impacts on family members' stress and well-being (e.g., Port, 2004). Similarly, recent work has suggested the considerable variability in adaptation of caregivers to bereavement; some studies have shown overall decreases in depression following bereavement (e.g., Schulz et al., 2003), and caregivers who indicate greater pre-loss benefit or "non-strain" associated with caregiving are more likely to report greater depression post-loss (Boerner, Schulz, & Horowitz, 2004).

LINKING LONGITUDINAL RESEARCH TO PRACTICE AND POLICY

As suggested in the summarization above, caregiving has a number of long-term effects on families and their disabled care recipients. This is particularly evident when considering the various transitions that may occur, such as assumption of care responsibilities, institutionalization, or bereavement. The existing mechanism designed to assist disabled older adults and their caregiving families is community-based long-term care (CBLTC), which includes a range of programs and services to: (1) address and alleviate the care needs of older persons in the community, and (2) in some instances, provide respite or relief to informal caregivers. The most prominent forms of CBLTC include in-home help (e.g., assistance with household chores, personal care, companion services) and adult day services (out-of-home services, such as therapeutic activities, health monitoring, socialization, medical care, and transportation for older adults with a variety of impairments). However, from the early 1980s to more recent efforts, it has been acknowledged that the provision of CBLTC to impaired older adults and their informal caregivers has mixed or no effects in immediately reducing stress or other negative caregiving outcomes (e.g., Gaugler & Zarit, 2001; Gottlieb & Johnson, 2000). Issues from liberal targeting to low service utilization often attenuated the potency of CBLTC, making it difficult to determine whether these programs could exert positive health benefits for informal caregivers or their elderly care recipients. Of those evaluations that did provide significant effects, most utilized small samples, had design intervals of 1-year or less, and implemented "per protocol" designs where participants were not randomly assigned to a treatment or control condition, thus increasing threats to internal validity.

Practice and Policy Recommendations

Support of Flexible Community-Based Long-Term Care. As existing longitudinal research on caregiving demonstrates, informal long-term care is a complex process that does not progress in a uniform manner. In addition to the considerable increases, decreases, or stability that caregivers may indicate on key psychosocial outcomes, caregivers can also experience a number of transitions at markedly diverse time points throughout their caregiving careers. While program flexibility has long been emphasized by researchers and practitioners alike (Montgomery & Kosloski, 2000), several questions emerge about how to achieve flexible alternative modes of service delivery in CBLTC. Do policies and support programs exist that consider the heterogeneity of caregivers when administering appropriate support programs? Similarly, do respite or psychosocial programs for families acknowledge the diverse histories or trajectories of the caregiving experience prior to intake or initial service utilization? A policy recommendation that is by no means unique to this paper is that acknowledging the diversity of caregiving families via policies that support flexible targeting and delivery of traditional CBLTC services may improve the overall impact of these programs.

Several recent policy initiatives have demonstrated some degree of success when moving beyond traditional models of CBLTC delivery and creating more flexible support for families, and thus serve as policy models for any future demonstration efforts. For example, the Alzheimer's Disease Demonstration Grants to States (ADDGS) was authorized in 1990 by Congress via the Public Health Services Act (Public Law 101-557) and has been reauthorized three times. Now administered by the Administration on Aging, the ADDGS' main objective is to enhance and develop statewide support services for persons with Alzheimer's disease and their caregivers. ADGGS annual funding through

2002 was at 11.5 million dollars, and the grants were awarded on a competitive basis to 11 states (Montgomery, 2002). A major emphasis of the ADDGS was program flexibility; communities were encouraged not only to create new services, but also to adapt and refine existing models of support that enhance current approaches to Alzheimer's care in the community. As noted by Starns (2002) in a policy review of the ADDGS, several states made notable strides in refining existing CBLTC programs. For example, to address some of the traditional barriers of rural and low-income communities such as workforce shortages and lack of reliable transportation, Georgia has developed a mobile adult day program that provides traditional adult day services at various sites, as needed, in communities that could not afford a full-time adult day facility. Transportation was arranged for disabled older adults through existing community support resources. Maine created teams of evaluators (each team consisted of a social worker and nurse) to conduct home visits, consult with geriatric physicians, and develop individualized care plans. As the only evaluation program available for rural older adults in northeastern Maine, the program has reached a considerable number of cognitively impaired older adults and family members who would otherwise not receive traditional CBLTC services.

Another example of service flexibility is the Cash and Counseling Demonstration and Evaluation (CCDE). The CCDE is perhaps one the most flexible service options available to older consumers in need of care in the community. It currently provides Medicaid consumers in three states (Florida, Arkansas, and New Jersey) a cash allowance as well as informational support, in contrast to agency-based models that typify most CBLTC services (Simon-Rusinowitz, Mahoney, Loughlin, & DeBarthe Sadler, 2005). Consumers are allowed to use the cash allowance to purchase not only in-home care and support, but also assistive devices or other options (e.g., home modifications). Information services provide consumers with training in hiring, retention, payment, and management of care providers. The CCDE is supported under 1115 Research and Demonstration Waivers granted by the Center for Medicare and Medicaid Services.

Preliminary evaluation data from the Arkansas site suggest that the flexibility offered by cash and counseling may have a number of benefits for older consumers and their family caregivers, including the opportunity for family caregivers to strike a greater balance between work and care responsibilities, the ability of paid family caregivers to contribute to Social Security retirement and disability benefits, and supplementation of existing informal care (as opposed to "substitution," where publicly-reimbursed care replaces unpaid informal care; Simon-Rusin-owitz et al., 2005). Reductions in unmet need as well as high satisfaction on the part of cash and counseling consumers appear to add further support to the considerable flexibility consumer-directed approaches may offer. Prior policy concerns, such as quality of paid care provided by family members, inappropriate use of the cash option, reductions in labor supply for long-term care workers (e.g., nursing aides), and increased strain on the part of directly hired workers did not emerge in the preliminary evaluation of the Arkansas CCDE data (see also Dale, Brown, Phillips, & Carlson, 2005). Other recent evaluation data from the Arkansas CCDE suggested that, after 10 months, informal caregivers spent less time providing care assistance to older adults in the CCDE treatment condition. In addition, informal caregivers in the CCDE treatment group indicated greater satisfaction with care arrangements and indicated less social, emotional, or physical strain than controls (Foster, Brown, Phillips, & Lepidus Carlson, 2005). Other findings demonstrated the costs implication of cash and counseling services; while CCDE clients reported higher Medicaid personal care expenses than controls during the first year of enrollment, these costs were offset in the following year since clients in the CCDE utilized less nursing home care and other Medicaid-reimbursed services (Dale, Brown, Phillips, Schore, & Carlson, 2003).

When taking longitudinal caregiving research into account, it is clear that these exemplar approaches may have similar success in addressing diverse needs not only *across* families, but also *within* families over time. Given the complexities of impending health-related transitions, policies that can mandate flexible programming and services that not only assist families caring for loved ones at-home but also following institutionalization or similar transitions could offer more wide-ranging benefits than have been realized within existing service networks.

Timing of Delivery. Some evidence suggests that CBLTC utilization earlier in the dementia caregiving career may yield more substantial benefits for disabled older adults and their family caregivers. Emerging research has begun to analyze the long-term challenges facing those individuals who recently assume care responsibilities. The admittedly few existing findings imply that, in contrast to wear and tear conceptualizations of adaptation (where caregiver stress and other negative outcomes exacerbate over time; see Townsend, Noelker, Deimling, & Bass, 1989), those individuals in the earlier stages of caregiving may experience increased stress and depression in both general and dementia-specific informal care contexts (Burton et al., 2003; Gaugler, Kane et al., 2005b; Gaugler, Zarit, & Pearlin et al., 2003a). To some extent, the descriptive and/or exploratory findings potentially support the need to deliver CBLTC services that provide respite earlier in the dementia caregiving career, as the demands and events that occur soon after caregiving onset may precipitate negative caregiving outcomes.

The key implication in this discussion of timing is that eligibility for CBLTC and similar services is often restricted or limited for those with serious functional or cognitive dependencies. Unfortunately, this may also mean that there is nearly total reliance on informal/family care-givers prior to eligibility for publicly-funded CBLTC, particularly for those families who do not have reliable access to private-pay sources of formal services. It is possible that relaxing eligibility criteria for dis-abled older adults and their families in order to intervene earlier in the caregiving career may result in a significant expansion of public fund-ing, and is thus a serious public policy constraint. However, as current research suggests, in instances where CBLTC is utilized for potentially overburdened caregivers earlier in their respective care trajectories, there is also the possibility for reduced public spending as these individ-uals may maintain their informal caregiving roles longer than if no for-mal assistance is provided (Gaugler et al., 2005b). Although few studies have directly tested whether the timing of service use within the infor-mal care context is associated with reducing negative caregiving out-comes over time, it is an area of research that may have some degree of policy import.

Program Content and Targeting. Advances in longitudinal research outline several policy strategies to enhance the content and targeting of CBLTC services. As some researchers suggest, long-term care policies providing financial support to CBLTC services should emphasize im-provements in program content to impact health outcomes more di-rectly (e.g., Gaugler & Zarit, 2001; Henry & Reifler, 1997). This is particularly apparent when considering the longitudinal characteristics and progression of informal long-term care; as opposed to more static, uniform types of service provision that only focus on the disabled el-derly client, policies and programs that incorporate the changing needs . of caregiving families may be desirable. For example, many adult day programs do not remain open on weekends or evenings to meet care-givers' and clients' needs (Henry & Reifler, 1997). Outreach efforts that incorporate the concerns of informal care providers and consider the changing needs and dynamics of family care over time when refining their service would be an ideal starting point for new and innovative policy initiatives.

A good example of how current policy may disallow content flexibility to meet the needs of informal caregivers over time is Medicare policy. For some CBLTC services to remain eligible for Medicare funding, they must conform to a health model of service provision (for example, limited rehabilitative therapies, intravenous medications, etc.). While this means a greater proportion of Medicare dollars may flow toward CBLTC services such as adult day programs, this may restrict overall choice, eligibility, access, and, perhaps most importantly, flexibility in program content to address the needs not only of clients in various stages of chronic disease (such as dementia) but the diverse needs of informal long-term care providers. For example, as a review of the adult day service literature emphasizes, medicalized models of adult day care do not provide significantly greater benefits to elderly clients or their caregivers when compared to more "social" models of care (Gaugler & Zarit, 2001). In this instance, federal regulations and the reimbursement attached to them may hinder the ability of various CBLTC programs to deliver or offer sensitive, flexible benefits to caregivers over time. It should be noted, however, that this recommendation reflects a major shift in Medicare policy, particularly in light of the 1997 Balanced Budget Act that emphasized Medicare's place as a source of payment for acute care, and not chronic disease management or long-term care. However, given the need for integration of reimbursement sources to meet the needs of chronically disabled older adults and their informal caregivers, creating more flexible modes of public reimbursement may prove necessary as the U.S. population continues to age, particularly among the oldest-old age group (i.e., 85 years of age and over; see www.census.gov).

Another policy issue that is informed by longitudinal research on caregiving is targeting. Some of the available longitudinal research on informal long-term care suggests that targeting of services may be more effective when the focus moves beyond the older adult and incorporates several elements of the caregiving process, including caregiver burden and timing (i.e., helping those who have recently begun to assume care responsibilities intensively and then providing more sustained but less intensive support throughout the subsequent stages of care; see Gaugler, Zarit et al., 2003a). By considering elements of the informal caregiving system, policies that support CBLTC to prevent caregiver distress or other costly outcomes may offer more integrative programs that can alleviate the diverse needs and challenges of family care providers.

Additional guidance on the targeting of services to meet the needs of caregivers at diverse points in their respective careers is provided by Montgomery and Kosloski (2000). As the authors emphasize, caregivers will likely not access or utilize services if there is no perceived need, or costs (whether they be financial, psychological, or functional/ physical) outweigh potential benefits from the perspective of the caregiver. In response, Montgomery and Kosloski (2000) forward several practice recommendations designed to improve the targeting of services through the following program modalities (pp. 162-165):

1. *Education.* For education to exert the greatest benefit, the information provided must match the needs of the caregiver as well as that caregiver's position in his or her respective career. For example, in earlier stages of caregiving, families may be most likely to seek information about the disease process (such as dementia or Alzheimer's disease), what services are available, and the legal and financial ramifications of care provision. However, as the potential stress and psychological manifestations of care provision take shape over time, later-stage caregivers may require more specific information on care management skills and available support. When care-related transitions are impending, such as nursing home placement, education must emphasize the nature of residential long-term care, ways to promote effective involvement in facility care routines, and outlets for family advocacy. Unlike other strategies, which tend to emphasize generalized dissemination approaches, the information delivered must consider each individual's caregiving career.

2. *Support groups.* As with educational approaches, caregivers may experience various benefits from support groups due to diversity in context (e.g., spouse vs. adult child; time point in the caregiving career). Whereas spousal support groups may benefit participants by allowing the opportunity to discuss relationship issues and encourage help-seeking behaviors, adult child support groups may prove most successful when focusing on the expansion of participants' support network and information related to the disease process. Similar diversity of experience (and benefit) may extend to caregivers in the early, middle, or later stages of their caregiving careers, or caregivers who have experienced different transitions, such as onset, institutionalization, or bereavement. Creating poli-

cies and programs that offer support group modules that are sensitive to this contextual diversity (as opposed to a one-size-fits-all approach) are likely to exert more positive benefits than have been demonstrated in the current literature.

3. *Respite.* Although the findings on the effectiveness of case management, adult day services, and in-home help have been mixed, there is evidence to suggest that underutilization of CBLTC services, coupled with a lack of understanding for how clients actually use available services, may help to explain the lack of benefits. There are likely differences in how various family caregivers utilize CBLTC (e.g., spouses may not identify themselves as caregivers until late in the disease process, resulting in delayed utilization, while adult child caregivers who provide support in earlier stages of the disease may not perceive a need for such support). Due to these variations in the caregiving career, the delay of CBLTC use occurs, limiting the efficacy of these services to improve caregiving outcomes (Gaugler, Kane et al., 2005b). Considering the dyadic relationship between the caregiver and care recipient, cultural factors, and the point where individuals identify themselves as caregivers as well as the appropriate intensity (or, "dosage") and continuity of support will likely improve the benefits of respite services.

CONCLUSION

Although the provision of informal long-term care by families often occurs over prolonged periods of time, descriptive and/or exploratory research that captures the longitudinal aspects of family caregiving is relatively nascent. Perhaps one of the more promising avenues of research inquiry in family caregiving is the analysis of trajectories and transitions in family caregiving. Linking policy initiatives and program design to some of these key emerging findings may lead to considerable improvement in areas such as the flexibility, timing, and targeting of CBLTC delivery. By moving beyond the conceptualization of informal long-term care as a static event and instead reorienting policy initiatives to consider family caregiving as a career, services emerging from such approaches may hold considerable promise for alleviating the complex and multifaceted challenges disabled older people and their families now face.

AUTHOR NOTES

Joseph E. Gaugler, PhD, is Assistant Professor at the Center on Aging, Center for Gerontological Nursing, School of Nursing, the University of Minnesota. He can be contacted at the School of Nursing, University of Minnesota, 6-150 Weaver-Densford Hall, 1331, Minneapolis, MN 55455 (E-mail: gaug0015@umn.edu).

Pamela Teaster, PhD, is Assistant Professor at the Graduate Center in Gerontology, College of Public Health, University of Kentucky.

REFERENCES

Boerner, K., Schulz, R., & Horowitz, A. (2004). Positive aspects of caregiving and adaptation to bereavement. *Psychology and Aging, 19*: 668-675.

Burton, L. C., Zdaniuk, B., Schulz, R., Jackson, S., & Hirsch, C. (2003). Transitions in spousal caregiving. *The Gerontologist, 43*: 230-241.

Dale, S., Brown, R., Phillips, B., Schore, J., & Carlson, B. L. (2003). The effects of cash and counseling on personal care services and Medicaid costs in Arkansas. *Health Affairs, W3*: 566-575.

Dale, S., Brown, R., Phillips, B., & Carlson, B. L. (2005). How do hired workers fare under consumer-directed personal care? *The Gerontologist, 45*: 583-592.

Foster, L., Brown, R., Phillips, B., & Carlson, B. L. (2005). Easing the burden of caregiving: The impact of consumer direction on primary informal caregivers in Arkansas. *The Gerontologist, 45*: 474-485.

Gaugler, J. E., Kane, R. L., Kane, R. A., Clay, T., & Newcomer, R. (2003). Predicting institutionalization of cognitively impaired older people: Utilizing dynamic predictors of change. *The Gerontologist, 43*: 219-229.

Gaugler, J. E., Kane, R. L., Kane, R. A., & Newcomer, R. (2005a). The longitudinal influence of early behavior problems in the dementia caregiving career. *Psychology and Aging, 20*: 100-116.

Gaugler, J. E., Kane, R. L., Kane, R. A., & Newcomer, R. (2005b). Early community-based service utilization and its effects on institutionalization in dementia caregiving. *The Gerontologist, 45*: 177-185.

Gaugler, J. E., & Zarit, S. H. (2001). The effectiveness of adult day services for disabled older people. *Journal of Aging & Social Policy, 12*: 23-47.

Gaugler, J. E., Zarit, S. H., & Pearlin, L. I. (2003). The onset of dementia caregiving and its longitudinal implications. *Psychology and Aging, 18*: 171-180.

Gottlieb, B. H., & Johnson, J. (2000). Respite programs for caregivers of persons with dementia: A review with practice implications. *Aging and Mental Health, 4*(2): 119-129.

Henry, R. S., & Reifler, B. V. (1997). Coverage of adult day service in long-term care insurance policies. *Journal of Applied Gerontology, 16*(2): 221-234.

Lawton, M. P., Moss, M., Hoffman, C., & Perkinson, M. (2000). Two transitions in the daughter's caregiving careers. *The Gerontologist, 40*(4): 437-448.

Montgomery, R. J. V. (2002). Introduction: A new look at community-based respite programs: Utilization, satisfaction, and development. *Home Health Care Services Quarterly, 21:* 1-4.

Montgomery, R. J. V., & Kosloski, K. D. (2000). Family caregiving: Change, continuity, and diversity. In M. P. Lawton, & R. L. Rubenstein (Eds.), *Interventions in dementia care: Toward improving quality of life* (pp. 143-171). New York, NY: Springer.

Montgomery, R. J. V., & Williams, K. N. (2001). Implications of differential impacts of caregiving for future research on Alzheimer's care. *Aging and Mental Health, 5:* S23-S35.

Pavalko, E. K., & Woodbury, S. (2000). Social roles as process: Caregiving careers and women's health. *Journal of Health and Social Behavior, 41:* 91-105.

Pearlin, L. I. (1992). The careers of caregivers. *The Gerontologist, 32:* 647.

Pearlin, L. I., & Aneshensel, C. S. (1994). Caregiving: The unexpected career. *Social Justice Research, 7:* 373-390.

Pearlin, L. I., Lieberman, M., Menaghan, E., & Mullan, J. (1981). The stress process. *Journal of Health and Social Behavior, 22:* 337-356.

Port, C. L. (2004). Identifying changeable barriers to family involvement in the nursing home for cognitively impaired residents. *The Gerontologist, 44:* 770-778.

Roth, D., Haley, W., Owen, J., Clay, O., & Goode, K. (2001). Latent growth models of the longitudinal effects of dementia caregiving: A comparison of African-American and White family caregivers. *Psychology and Aging, 16:* 427-436.

Schulz, R., Belle, S. H., Czaja, S. J., McGinnis, K. A., Stevens, A., & Zhang, S. (2004). Long-term care placement of dementia patients and caregiver health and well-being. *Journal of the American Medical Association, 292:* 961-967.

Schulz, R., Mendelsohn, A. B., Haley, W. E., Mahoney, D., Allen, R. S., Zhang, S., Thompson, L., & Belle, S. H. (2003). End-of-life care and the effects of bereavement on family caregivers of persons with dementia. *New England Journal of Medicine, 349:* 1936-1942.

Simon-Rusinowitz, L., Mahoney, K. J., Loughlin, D. M., & Debarthe Sadler. (2005). Paying family caregivers: An effective policy option in the Arkansas Cash and Counseling Demonstration. *Marriage & Family Review, 37:* 83-105.

Starns, M. K. (2002). Comment on the utility of the ADDGS Evaluation for policy and practice. *Home Health Care Services Quarterly, 21:* 133-139.

Townsend, A., Noelker, L., Deimling, G., & Bass, D. (1989). Longitudinal impact of interhousehold caregiving on adult children's mental health. *Psychology and Aging, 4:* 393-401.

Vitaliano, P. P., Zhang, J., & Scanlan, J. M. (2003). Is caregiving hazardous to one's physical health? A meta-analysis. *Psychological Bulletin, 129:* 946-972.

Yamamoto, M. N., Aneshensel, C. S., & Levy-Storms, L. (2002). Patterns of family visiting with institutionalized elders: The case of dementia. *Journals of Gerontology: Psychological Sciences, 57:* S234-S246.

doi:10.1300/J031v18n03_10

Zoning, Accessory Dwelling Units, and Family Caregiving: Issues, Trends, and Recommendations

Phoebe S. Liebig, PhD
Teresa Koenig, MSG
Jon Pynoos, PhD

University of Southern California

SUMMARY. This article explores the relationship between zoning regulations and co-residential family caregiving in the United States. It first provides an overview of U.S. housing policies, especially zoning. We then describe major changes in family structure and composition in the United States with their implications for caregiving and discuss how multigenerational housing options, particularly accessory dwelling units (ADUs) in single-family homes, can help support family caregiving. After an overview of zoning policies and actions that inhibit ADU production, we document current trends, incorporating information from a small non-random study of ADU activity we conducted in 2004. Finally, we present recommendations for promoting more multigenerational housing as a supplement to other family support programs (e.g., dependent care assistance, family caregiver payments) and as a source of affordable, supportive housing for those families choosing co-residence as their eldercare solution. doi:10.1300/J031v18n03_11 *[Article copies available for a fee from The Haworth Document Delivery Service: 1-800-HAWORTH. E-mail address: <docdelivery@haworthpress.com> Website: <http://www.HaworthPress.com> © 2006 by The Haworth Press, Inc. All rights reserved.]*

[Haworth co-indexing entry note]: "Zoning, Accessory Dwelling Units, and Family Caregiving: Issues, Trends, and Recommendations." Liebig, Phoebe S., Teresa Koenig, and Jon Pynoos. Co-published simultaneously in *Journal of Aging & Social Policy* (The Haworth Press, Inc.) Vol. 18, No. 3/4, 2006, pp. 155-172; and: *Family and Aging Policy* (ed: Francis G. Caro) The Haworth Press, Inc., 2006, pp. 155-172. Single or multiple copies of this article are available for a fee from The Haworth Document Delivery Service [1-800-HAWORTH, 9:00 a.m. - 5:00 p.m. (EST). E-mail address: docdelivery@haworthpress. com].

KEYWORDS. Zoning, family caregiving, multigenerational housing, accessory dwelling units, co-residence

INTRODUCTION

American families, like their counterparts worldwide, provide the bulk of care for elders and other vulnerable family members, based on social norms, psychological preferences, and economic capacity. Public and private decision makers grapple with how best to support families in their caregiving roles at a time when the American family has undergone significant structural changes and the need for long-term care has increased due to greater longevity of the general population and of those with a disability acquired earlier in life. However, U.S. housing policy, in comparison with western European and Asian nations, has rarely been seen as a strategy to enhance family support of elders (Liebig, 2001). Instead, post-World War II housing and tax policies at the national and state levels have promoted the American dream: owner-occupied, single-family detached homes for nuclear families in the suburbs (Pynoos & Redfoot, 1995; Duany, Plater-Zyberk, & Speck, 2000; Hayden, 2003). Local land-use policies, framed by zoning ordinances emphasizing single use, a distinctly American planning concept, have been enacted to protect the integrity and value of residential neighborhoods against commercial and industrial activities (Duany et al., 2000; Hayden, 2003).

However, these zoning practices have resulted in poor access to services, particularly in suburban areas that rely heavily or exclusively on private automobiles, and also have led to restrictions on expanding or altering family homes that could provide more affordable housing and promote/support family caregiving, while enhancing the privacy, independence, and safety of elders. To meet these challenges, strategies have included the development of home- and community-based services, tax incentives for dependent care, and the National Family Caregiver Support Program. Generally overlooked in mainstream discussions about supporting family caregivers, however, are the regulatory barriers to creating multigenerational, family-based supportive housing, for example, accessory dwelling units in single-family homes.

Today, 13% of all elders live with relatives other than a spouse (Pynoos & Golant, 1995), as do about one-fourth of those aged 85 (Linsk & Keigher, 1995). This proportion is likely to grow, given the phenomenon of boomerang parents who return to live near or with their children when they become frail or economically overextended. In addition, the preferences of Asian and Hispanic immigrants for living in multigenerational households (Burr & Mutchler, 1993) will likely drive an increased demand for housing that accommodates those desires. For the most part, however, zoning policies are stuck in the mid-20th century and are not in synch with the changing demographics of age and American family composition or the growing need for long-term care.

U.S. HOUSING POLICY AND ZONING REGULATION: AN OVERVIEW

Modern U.S. housing policy essentially began at the turn of the 20th century. Two global wars and the Great Depression softened the stance against federal interventions. Unlike European policies centered on building and/or managing public housing, the emphasis was on promoting home ownership, the American dream (Pynoos & Liebig, 1995; Pynoos & Redfoot, 1995). The ideal of a single-family dwelling designed for a married couple with their children allowed Americans to establish households that afforded them privacy and separateness from others, such as their parents, siblings, or other relatives. By the 1930s, the loosening of kin networks by single-family housing became accepted as the norm (Hayden, 2003: 118). This contrasted with advertisements of the late 1890s and early 1900s for suburban housing showing a male owner, surrounded by his wife and children and an elderly female (Hayden, 2003: 82); the patterns of religious groups, such as the Mormons, Amish, and Mennonites, who housed their elders within the family home; or the existence of family compounds or clusters, often found in 19th century New England and the Middle West.

The 1920s set the stage for local zoning practices. The national Standard Zoning Enabling Act of 1923 set forth a uniform policy empowering each state to structure the power to zone and delegate that power to municipalities (Pollak, 1994). It subsequently served as a template for enabling acts in all 50 states. Three years later, the U.S. Supreme Court ruled in *Village of Euclid v. Amber Realty* that zoning ordinances and regulations would be presumed to be legal until challenged successfully in the courts. The challenger would have to prove a personally deleterious impact of the contested zoning law (Pollak & Gorman, 1989; Golant, 1992). For the next 50 years, this landmark decision undergirded exclusionary zoning practices across the nation, with both states and local governments playing major roles in regulation and its enforcement. Judicial review of local ordinances continued to be a major factor in the implementation of zoning laws.

The Euclid case essentially codified the zoning practices of the early 1900s. The U.S. exploitation of land as a commodity, aimed at maximizing resale value rather than its value for long-term use within a community, led to zoning codes that separated homes, shops, and offices (Pollak & Gorman, 1989; Pindell, 1995). Model zoning ordinances were generated to rationalize land use, so local governments could restrict population and structural densities. The separate zoning of single-family residences away from multi-family dwellings was a means of drawing lines between the sizes and types of families living in suburbs and urban areas (Gellen, 1985; Hayden, 2003; Liberty, 2003).

With these barriers firmly in place, it was virtually impossible for developers, builders, or multigenerational families to penetrate residential neighborhoods zoned for single-family housing with any alternative design, such as accessory dwelling units (ADUs), at least not legally. Zoning ordinances screened out these nonconforming structures via complex development and construction standards that often rendered a project fiscally prohibitive. Definitions of the type of family eligible to reside in single-family homes also were written into zoning ordinances, thereby codifying the traditional family as a two-generational unit composed of a husband, wife, and their children. Regulations excluded households composed of persons unrelated by blood, such as students, families with foster children, group homes for persons with mental or physical disabilities, and even elders and their live-in caretakers (Pollak & Gorman, 1989). Local ordinances operating within the framework of each state's precedents, enabling laws, and constitutional protections were, over time, incorporated into national housing policies, adding a federal layer of statutes and protections (Pollak & Gorman, 1989).

Several U.S. housing policies of the 1930s and 1940s, for example, the Federal Home Loan Bank Act, the Housing Act of 1937, and the GI Bill at the end of World War II, led to expanded home ownership, the primary goal of U.S. housing policy (Pynoos & Redfoot, 1995). By 1950, more than half of American families owned their homes (U.S. Census Bureau, 2001a). Few retirement communities existed, largely because they were not needed. Elders stayed in their old inner city neighborhoods as their adult children scattered into the new suburbs; if unable to drive, they could maintain a viable lifestyle by walking (Duany et al., 2000; Hayden, 2003).

Today's elders, the suburban in-movers of the post-World War II period, have been major beneficiaries of these policies; their levels of home ownership (77%) are highest for all age groups (Pynoos & Redfoot, 1995). However, the desire of today's elders to age in place in suburbia is compromised by the lack of adequate transportation and walkability and the strict separation of land uses accomplished by zoning ordinances. Accessing needed services requires greater effort by older adults (and their family caregivers), as well as other victims of suburban sprawl, such as bored teenagers and weary commuters (Duany et al., 2000: 115-135). In many ways, single-family housing is less likely to meet the changing needs of the households and family structures that have evolved over the past half century (Sickle & Kascal, 1984).

THE CHANGING AMERICAN FAMILY, LIVING ARRANGEMENTS, AND ELDER CARE

The traditional American family envisioned by the zoning laws of the first half of the 20th century has changed in several ways: structure, ethnicity, and longevity, with implications for living arrangements and eldercare. In 1988, married couples with children constituted 27% of all households; only 8.8% were composed of the ideal family of a male breadwinner, stay at home wife, and two children (Pollak & Gorman, 1989). By 2000, only 24% of the nation's 105 million households could be defined as traditional families (Cobb & Dvorak, 2000).

American family composition has become more diverse and smaller; young singles and older persons living alone have become a dominant group (Hayden, 2003). Between 1970 and 2000, families of only one or two persons increased from 46% to 58.6%. Those with four to five members decreased from 36.7% to 25%, with the average size of the American family declining from 3.14 to 2.62 persons (U.S. Census, 2001b). Households increasingly include married couples without children, non-related persons (intentional families) or unmarried partners (Cobb & Dvorak, 2000; U.S. Census, 2001b). Furthermore, more women working outside the home and a higher proportion of marriages ending in divorce and often remarriage have led to more dual-earner, single-parent, and blended families. One outcome of these changes is fewer family members are available to provide eldercare.

The American family also has become more diverse ethnically and racially. Immigration, especially from Latin America and Asia, has changed the face of the U.S. population. By 2000, racial and ethnic minorities were about 27% of the total population; by 2015, they will constitute one-third (Cutler & Hendricks, 2001). In just two decades, minorities will add 25.3 million to the total population, with Hispanics leading all other ethnic groups (Harvard Joint Center on Housing Studies, 2003). The proportion of minority persons aged 65 and older also will increase from 16% in 1998 to 24% in 2025, partly due to immigration–many arrived in this country when they were 55 or older (Cutler & Hendricks, 2001; Glick & Van Hook, 2002). Minority elders are more likely to live with their families, because they come from cultures based on kinship networks and co-residence (Wilmoth, 2001) and may derive social and economic support from their children (Glick & Van Hook, 2002). Within the next 20 years, the preferences of minorities, middle-aged or older singles, and empty-nesters will shape housing demands (Harvard Joint Center on Housing Studies, 2003).

Another factor affecting the American family has been increased longevity. Family age structure has changed from a pyramid, characteristic of early 20th century families, to a beanpole, reflecting a family with more generations, but with fewer members in each generation. The resulting multigenerational family experiences longer years of shared life, with grandparents and other kin available to participate in family functions and responsibilities (Bengtson, 2001).

This structural change has occurred at the same time that federal and state policies are cutting back on many social welfare programs; families increasingly will be called upon to fill the resulting gaps as governments reduce their fiscal commitment to welfare, caregiving, and well-being expenditures (Bengtson, 2001; Bengtson, Lowenstein, Putney, & Gans, 2003). Of the estimated 23 million caregiving households, approximately 21% have either a co-residing elderly spouse, parent, relative, or friend (National Alliance for Caregiving and AARP, 1997). It is clear that American families are willing and able to care for their older family members, often by co-residing. For many, multigenerational housing in single-family homes, for example, accessory dwelling units (ADUs), is a viable, often preferred care alternative to board and care homes, continuing-care retirement communities, or nursing homes. In addition, intergenerational co-residence can be a solution to the growing lack of affordable housing for both younger and older households.

Beyond these considerations, co-residential housing can strengthen family ties and promote age integration, important social policy goals. Grandparents in the home can share parenting responsibilities and ease tensions between parents and their children, decrease involvement in delinquent activities, reduce depressive episodes, and improve children's academic performance (Uhlenberg, 2000). The proximity of grandparents and other elderly relatives affords children and adolescents an opportunity to share in caregiving activities, while learning empathy, compassion, and the value of service to others. Other benefits of multigenerational housing include increasing generational solidarity to help erode ageism and the resentment younger cohorts often express in generational equity debates (Uhlenberg, 2000).

The elderly feel safer, more secure, and less socially isolated with family members readily accessible. Adult children or other relatives are less anxious about the well-being of their elders because they can interact with them daily on a face-to-face basis, while the younger generation's computer skills can help their elders in gaining desired information and maintaining contact with friends and other family members (Pollak, 1994; Uhlenberg, 2000). Multigenerational living arrangements can help elders maintain a sense of independence and autonomy while easing their adjustment back into the larger family environment when they are less able to care for themselves (Cobb & Dvorak, 2000). They also can facilitate aging in place in the homes to which elders have strong emotional attachments, while at the same time providing an affordable place for younger family members to live (Gellen, 1985).

MULTIGENERATIONAL HOUSING: CO-HOUSING, SHARED HOUSING, ACCESSORY DWELLING UNITS

One solution to meet the demographic challenges and housing issues noted in this article is to create more multigenerational housing that meets privacy needs of older and younger family members, while enhancing the security and independence of elders. One, often costly, approach is building new, affordable housing to accommodate multigenerational caregiving families. But the use/conversion of existing single-family residences is an efficient alternative (Nelson, 2003).

Multigenerational housing encompasses co-housing, shared housing, and accessory dwelling units (ADUs). All help expand the supply of affordable housing, enhance family solidarity, and ensure that elders have a supportive environment, with security and services provided by their families, however family is defined. Co-housing and shared housing, relatively recent phenomena, are usually associated with intentional or voluntary families not composed of persons related by blood or marriage. By contrast, ADUs are focused on kinship families and are not a new idea, having been in existence since colonial days. They were popular up through the 1940s, before the era of suburbanization and the nuclear family (Cobb & Dvorak, 2000). Renewed interest surfaced in the1970s and 1980s, when a small number of developers believed they could build ADUs for a price below the normal per-resident land costs and offer affordable, supportive housing to the older market (Folts & Muir, 2002).

Co-housing, initiated in Denmark in the late 1960s, was adopted in America in the late 1980s. A type of intentional community, it houses its residents in private homes–typically 40 units–with full kitchens, along with extensive common facilities: a common dining room and central kitchen, meeting rooms, lounges, libraries, workshops and play areas for children (McCamant & Durret, 1988). These homes can include flexible spaces: separate, private units to accommodate older relatives or be used by owners at a later stage of their own lives. Subject to the agreements made by the co-housing community, as well as local zoning laws, some have supplementary rooms (S rooms) located in the common area to be used by guests or rented by a family needing separate space for a relative, such as a teenager or older family member. However, co-housing in America has been limited due to land costs and zoning.

Shared housing is an agency-sponsored activity that provides help in structuring communal living in a single-family residence, offering individuals an opportunity to reduce housing costs, meet social needs, be more secure, and retain independence within a supportive environment. *Match programs* help identify home owners with excess space, often older adults, to locate compatible sharers; program success has usually depended on an intergenerational approach (Sickle & Kascal, 1984). However, programs are difficult to maintain due to funding problems and finding unrelated persons willing to assume greater care responsibilities as elderly occupants experience more health problems. *Shared group residences*, often intergenerational, are exemplified by the Shared Living House in Boston, a home for 14 persons aged 20 to 80 making joint decisions about the house and its functions (Sickle & Kascal, 1984). Similar programs have been created elsewhere, but zoning language limiting the number of unrelated persons who can be recognized as a family and classifying these residences as boarding or rooming homes have been major stumbling blocks to their widespread development.

Accessory dwellings units (ADU) comprise several categories: mother-in-law apartment, granny flat, elder cottage, carriage house, or garage apartment, but they share common attributes. They are residential units that provide independent living facilities for one or more persons, with designated areas for cooking and sanitation, plus space for living, sleeping and eating. They can be attached to or detached from another residence and located on the same parcel of land as the primary single-family home they accompany (Hare & Overton, 1993; Pollak, 1994). While these subcategories are often used interchangeably, each term has a distinct meaning (Pollak, 1994).

The accessory or mother-in-law apartment is created within an existing single-family home, utilizing available spare space (e.g., basement, attic), or by adding a new unit onto either an existing or new single-family residence. It has its own kitchen and bathroom; privacy is provided by a door that closes and locks separating it from the principal dwelling. This approach is different from housing an elder in an existing bedroom/den because it has separate, rather than shared, cooking and bathing facilities and affords greater privacy to all family members.

An accessory cottage is a separate, permanent structure placed on the same parcel or lot as the single-family home. While it can be an attached or detached structure, it is not built within the existing primary dwelling. Accessory cottages are also known as guest cottages or carriage houses. Garage or barn apartments are similar entities because they are not part of the primary dwelling; the latter is more popular in rural areas.

ECHO housing, or Elder Cottage Housing Opportunity housing, first created in Australia in the 1970s, is also known as a granny flat or elder cottage. ECHO housing refers to small, detached living units usually placed to the side or in back of the principal dwelling on the same lot, enabling adult children to care for their aging parent(s) and other older relatives. Often prefabricated units, ECHO housing can, in most cases, be installed in a day, including electrical, water and sewer hookups, making them more affordable than other ADUs. About the size of a two-car garage, they often include a living room, bedroom, bathroom, kitchen, pantry and utility room, with suitable door clearances for wheelchairs (Hare, 1991). However, zoning restrictions require the removal of units when they are no longer needed; the attendant costs have been a major barrier to their usage (Hare, 1991; Hare & Overton, 1993).

Due to these and other exclusionary zoning practices, the single-family home has become less responsive to the changing realities of America's families. These regulations constitute the most powerful barrier to appropriate, accessible, and affordable housing for our aging population (Pollak & Gorman, 1989; Howe et al., 1994; Golant, 1992; Cobb & Dvorak, 2000; Liberty, 2003). Still, homeowners have continued to build ADUs that often are illegal or not up to code, a major concern of local policymakers. Between 65,000 and 300,000 units are created each year (Gellen, 1985; Cobb & Dvorak, 2000). Furthermore, neighbors raise concerns about ADUs becoming permanent rentals, thereby changing neighborhoods from single-family homes to multifamily dwellings and negatively impacting property values (Sickle & Kascal, 1984: 77). These expressions of NIMBY (Not In My Back Yard) also concern local policymakers.

Zoning Regulations and ADUs

Under the U.S. Constitution, the zoning police power is essentially reserved to the states, which have the authority to enforce conditions of land use and planning regulations to promote the public good and protect public health, safety, and welfare. City and county ordinances set forth consistent, appropriate, and planned land use patterns for a particular jurisdiction in its general plan. In keeping with state requirements, a locality's general plan characteristically includes land use, circulation, housing, conservation, open space, noise, safety, and other elements (Quang Do, 2002: 798-799). A specific local plan also is generated to define zoning, subdivisions, and public works projects; zoning divides a city into districts, each with different regulations to advance order, convenience, prosperity, and the general welfare (Quang Do, 2002: 799-800). Typical land uses comprise the size and percentage of a lot occupied by a structure, density, standards for building setbacks from the street, and off-street parking requirements.

Exceptions to zoning ordinances can be obtained to promote ADUs. These include (1) variances, (2) nonconforming use and (3) conditional use. Variances are in direct conflict with a district's zoning and are granted to the property, not to the user. They are allowed because strict compliance would constitute extreme hardship for the owner (Quang Do, 2002, 799). Nonconforming use applies to land uses that existed before a conflicting zoning policy was implemented; these often grandfather in existing ADUs that are otherwise illegal. Conditional use allows a particular land use to exist even if it is inconsistent with current zoning so as to provide flexibility; many ADUs are permitted under this exception. Nonconforming and conditional uses must be decided on a case-by-case basis, generally entailing a lengthy and often expensive process involving planning commissions or departments and the city council.

An alternative to these exceptions are conversions by right contained in ADU-specific ordinances, sometimes mandated by state enabling laws. Oregon, through its anti-exclusionary zoning policy enacted in 1973, provided for regional regulations permitting ADUs, and since 1982, California has required cities and counties to allow ADU development, with limits on local governments' ability to deny or place restrictions on such development. Since 1993, Washington has required any city of at least 20,000 residents to allow ADUs. In a unique approach, Massachusetts offers tax exemptions for persons who build ADUs for seniors age 60 +.

However, most U.S. localities have enacted fairly detailed restrictions. These can include: (1) occupancy restrictions, for example, denying occupancy to anyone but a family member or to seniors over a certain age; (2) homeowner eligibility, for example, requiring the homeowners to live on-site; (3) neighborhood preservation, for example, prohibiting exterior modification to the principal dwelling; (4) location restrictions, for example, permitting ADUs only in new developments or limiting their numbers in any one neighborhood; (5) space requirements, for example, requiring a minimum or maximum ADU square footage or minimum lot-size; (6) mandating a certain number of additional off-street parking places; and (7) requiring extensive procedures, for example, multiple public hearings, lengthy plan reviews (Cobb & Dvorak, 2000; Nelson, 2003).

To track current trends, we undertook a small five-month study of ADU activity. A list of 32 cities in 13 states was compiled via a review of the academic literature and popular press using multiple databases, for example, Lexis/Nexis, ProQuest, Social Science Citation Index, Ageline, JSTOR, and Dissertation Abstracts. Websites for state and local governments and housing, planning and policy research institutes were searched, and key informants were contacted by telephone and email. A four-page questionnaire was created, reviewed and subsequently amended, and then sent by regular mail and email to city planners, zoning officials, or directors of community development. The survey instrument focused on four areas: general information, factors affecting ADU development; types of mechanisms employed for creating ADUs; and future projections of ADU supply. Twenty-one (69%) usable responses from 11 states were completed, in some instances via a telephone interview. Four cities in two of the original 13 states (Connecticut and Florida) declined to participate, due to staff shortages. Responses from western states included California, Colorado, Oregon, and Washington; eastern states comprised Massachusetts, Maryland, New York, North Carolina, Pennsylvania, and Virginia. One state (Illinois) was from the Midwest. Nearly one-third of the responses came from California cities.

Despite the obvious limitations of this study, we were able to glean impressions about current trends and issues surrounding ADUs. Respondents revealed that ordinances are their most common mechanism for creating ADUs, followed by conditional use permits. The majority of the ordinances in these 21 cities were enacted and amended between 1983 and 2004, usually at the behest of city planning commissions or elected officials, rather than consumers or building professionals. The earliest law (1949) was enacted by a California city; four cities had each passed three ADU-related laws since 1983. The most common ADU types are accessory apartments, followed by granny flats and garage apartments. One Western city, with land available for new housing development, reported automatically approving builders' plans with garage apartments.

Major factors affecting ADU development were the need for affordable housing and seniors' and adult children's preferences for multigenerational housing. Real estate developers played a minor role, while state mandates were a primary factor for cities in Washington, Oregon, and California. Two Eastern cities suggested their activities were designed to rationalize, not promote, ADUs, by ensuring that more become legal/up to code or trying to reduce the numbers of conversions to rental units. Factors inhibiting ADUs were traffic/parking congestion, population density, and privacy issues; surprisingly, property values and NIMBYism were of less concern. The primary criteria for obtaining an ADU permit were conformance with city building codes, parking, aesthetic design, and on-site occupancy by the homeowner. Only one city distinguished between ADU-approval criteria for older and new neighborhoods.

Actions to promote ADUs included expedited review and/or elimination of reviews or hearings; density bonuses (an approach often used to promote affordable housing of other kinds); technical assistance (e.g., publicizing ADU criteria that lead to approval without a conditional use permit); and creating a demonstration program to determine the levels of political feasibility of promoting ADUs. Despite these approaches, significant growth in the numbers of ADUs within the next five years was not seen as likely. Only three cities predicted more than 100 new ADUs, including one California city that has undertaken a comprehensive ADU Development Program. One Eastern city reported that its major job was to legalize its 15,000 existing ADUs, with its projected growth rate contingent on the success of those efforts.

CONCLUSIONS
AND RECOMMENDATIONS FOR ADU EXPANSION

Given the discussion above, it would appear that ADUs are an issue that has gained momentum on the policy agendas of all levels of government for the last 20 to 30 years. In the 1970s and 1980s, states initiated enabling laws focused specifically on this topic, with some subsequent action by localities. In the 1990s, a federal Task Force on Regulatory Barriers to Affordable Housing recommended removing restrictions on accessory apartments to enable elders to age in place; and the HUD Security Plan for Older Adults proposed helping older adults to remain in their homes and connected to their families and communities, and expanding affordable housing for low-income elders; both can be accomplished by ADUs. Many organizations, such as the National Association of Counties, the American Planning Association, AARP, and Fannie Mae have promoted ADUs, including proposing model state laws and local ordinances to speed up the adoption process (see Cobb & Dvorak, 2000). The implications of the Olmstead decision about the need to provide least restrictive long-term care environments are another factor that could propel greater acceptance of ADUs.

In addition, older consumer interest appears to be increasing. In 1997, a nationwide housing preference survey of persons aged 50+ conducted by AARP revealed that 36% would consider modifying their homes to include an ADU if they need assistance as they grow older (Cobb & Dvorak, 2000). Several authors (see Pollak & Gorman, 1989; Hare & Overton, 1993; Howe et al., 1994) note that elderly homeowners are interested in ADUs as a way to use their primary asset to enhance their income and personal security. Given the presumed political clout of elders at the local level, especially when life style issues are involved (Andel & Liebig, 2002), one might posit greater receptivity to ADUs.

However, other forces are operative. Stories in the popular press (e.g., *Los Angeles Times, The Wall Street Journal, U.S. News &World Report*) often focus on disruptions occasioned by ADUs: people with alternative life styles, code violations, and additional strain on infrastructure (streets, utilities). A recent event in California may explain ongoing resistance. In 2004, a bill (AB2702) that built on existing ADU laws sought to create statewide standards, for example, allowing ADUs in all residential zones, with a minimum unit size of 550 square feet. The bill was vetoed by Governor Schwarzenegger, largely based on arguments raised by groups such as the state branch of the American Planning Association, the California State Association of Counties, and the League of California Cities about state attempts to limit local control.

Beyond intergovernmental relations, other policy agendas can conflict with promoting ADUs. For example, although affordable housing falls under the rubric of economic development, an important state and local policy goal, it can connote invasion by the homeless and other undesirables, as well as the infamous and costly failures of public housing (Nelson, 2003: 4). The protection of property values (and therefore property tax revenues) also is a major concern for subnational governments, especially when called upon to pay for more services for the elderly. Additionally, arguments that elders are deserving of differential treatment may not be as powerful as they have been in the past (Andel & Liebig, 2002).

Given these push-pull factors, what might advocates do to promote ADUs that offer some promise of making it easier for families to provide caregiving on a co-residential basis? Three actions can be undertaken: (1) get more local ADU ordinances passed; (2) remove or ameliorate existing barriers to ADUs; and (3) engage stakeholder organizations in promoting model ordinances and disseminating case studies of cities and states that have increased ADUs. To get more ordinances passed, advocates need to educate themselves about their local zoning laws and procedures and how model laws can be used within that context. They also need to take advantage of a growing phenomenon, the use of community planning forums (Pindell, 1995), and tie the issue of ADUs to broader concerns, for example, creation of livable or elder-friendly communities, improving density ratios (Liberty, 2003). Advocates for the elderly and persons with disabilities need to join forces in local task forces or coalitions to promote family-based supportive housing, such as ADUs.

Another area requiring advocacy is to remove or ameliorate regulatory barriers to ADUs within existing ordinances or conditional use procedures. This approach encompasses several actions, such as expedited reviews, streamlining the permitting process, and enhancing coordination of the application process among all relevant city departments. It also can include expanding definitions of family to conform to the needs of local families.

Advocates can also work with stakeholder organizations to promote the several kinds of model ordinances developed by Cobb and Dvorak (2000) and to disseminate case studies of cities and states that have successfully increased ADUs. These partners might include governmental groups, for example, the National Association of Counties and National

League of Cities, and organizations with concerns about family or elder welfare, for example, the National Association of Social Workers, state offices of the AARP and Alzheimer's Association, and local Area Agencies on Aging (AAAs) as part of their National Family Caregiver Support Program efforts. These attempts to influence policymaking may defuse the kind of opposition exhibited in California's recent attempt to expand statewide ADU mandates.

State and local governments also have roles to play in expanding ADUs. States can collect statewide data on local ADU developments, describe innovative approaches, and convene local policymakers to address statewide issues and concerns. A state website on ADUs can provide information to a wide range of interested parties, for example, local officials, developers, consumers, service providers. Local jurisdictions also have a role to play, such as publishing guidebooks to assist applicants (e.g., consumers, developers) seeking permits for legal ADUs. They also can put information in local papers, at local libraries, and on their websites to explain what homeowners must do to get an ADU permit, for example, permissible types, legalizing ADUs not conforming to codes. Because single-family homes designed for occupancy by families with children often present challenges to older, disabled persons (Howe et al., 1994), localities might also provide information about universal design features, for example, hand-held showers, that can be incorporated in ADUs to enhance eldercare.

Finally, advocates need to recast ADUs as a family caregiving issue. Although ADUs have been seen primarily as an affordable housing issue, they also are a family issue and an aging issue. Eldercare has become a major policy concern over the past 20-25 years, with a growing emphasis on finding nongovernmental and/or non-federal solutions with minimum public investment. Adding other policy approaches, such as overcoming regulatory barriers, to those existing, for example, dependent care assistance, family leave provisions, and family caregiver payments are necessary, given the changes in American families and the sheer numbers of elders needing long-term care by 2050. Co-residence is not and will not be an answer for all families with eldercare responsibilities; however, preparing for the age boom just around the corner requires that we examine more forcefully the role of single-family housing as a major strategy to address the needs of an aging society and of family caregivers.

AUTHOR NOTES

Phoebe S. Liebig, PhD, is Associate Professor of Gerontology and Public Administration at the University of Southern California. Dr. Liebig has published widely in journals such as *The Gerontologist,* the *Journal of Aging & Social Policy, Housing Policy Debate,* and *Journal of Housing for the Elderly,* has co-edited several books, including *An Aging India* and *Housing Frail Elders,* and is a recipient of AGHE's Clark Tibbitts award. Corresponding author Liebig can be contacted at Andrus Gerontology Center, University of Southern California, Los Angeles, CA 90089 (E-mail: liebig@usc.edu).

Jon Pynoos, PhD, is the UPS Foundation Professor of Gerontology, Policy, Planning and Development at the Andrus Gerontology Center of the University of Southern California. He is an expert on housing and aging in place. He has written and co-edited six books on housing and the elderly including *Linking Housing and Services for Older Adults, Housing the Aged,* and *Housing Frail Elders.*

Teresa Koenig, MSG, was research assistant at the University of Southern California when this paper was written. She is now an independent communications specialist consultant in St. George, Utah, working with the Andrus Gerontology Center at USC and a local hospital in Utah.

REFERENCES

Andel, R., & Liebig, P. S. (2002). The city of Laguna Woods: A case of senior power in local politics. *Research on Aging, 24*(1): 87-105.

Bengtson, V. L. (2001). Beyond the nuclear family: The increasing importance of multigenerational bonds. *Journal of Marriage and Family, 63*(1): 1-16.

Bengtson, V. L., Lowenstein, A., Putney, N. M., & Gans, D. (2003). Global aging and the challenge to families. In V.L. Bengtson and A. Lowenstein (Eds.), *Global aging and challenges to families.* New York: Aldine, DeGruyter.

Burr, J. A., & Mutchler, J. E. (1993). Ethnic living arrangements: Cultural convergence or cultural manifestation? *Social Forces, 72*: 169-179.

Cobb, R. L., & Dvorak, S. (2000). *Accessory dwelling units: Model state act and local ordinance.* Washington, DC: AARP Public Policy Institute.

Cutler, S. J., & Hendricks, J. (2001). Emerging social trends. In R. H. Binstock and L. K. George (Eds.). *Handbook of aging and the social sciences* (5th ed.). San Diego, CA: Academic Press.

Duany, A., Plater-Zyberk, E., & Speck, J. (2000). *Suburban nation: The rise of sprawl and the decline of the American dream.* New York: North Point Press.

Folts, W. E., & Muir, K. B. (2002). Housing for older adults: New lessons from the past. *Research on Aging, 24*(1): 10-28.

Gellen, M. (1985). *Accessory apartments in single-family housing.* New Brunswick, NJ: Rutgers Center for Urban Policy Research.

Glick, J. E., & Van Hook, J. (2002). Parents' co-residence with adult children: Can immigration explain racial and ethnic variation? *Journal of Marriage and Family 64*(2): 240-253.

Golant, S. M. (1992). *Housing America's elderly: Many possibilities/few choices.* Newbury Park, CA: Sage Publications.

Hare, P. H. (1991). The ECHO housing/granny flat experience in the United States. *Journal of Housing for the Elderly, 7*: 57-69.

Hare, P. H., & Overton, J. (Eds.) (1993). *Accessory units resource guide: The state of the art.* Los Angeles, CA: Andrus Gerontology Center, National Resource and Policy Center on Housing and Long-Term Care.

Harvard Joint Center for Urban Studies (2003). *The state of the nation's housing.* Retrieved December 2003 from http://www.jchs.harvard.edu.

Hayden, D. (2003). *Building suburbia.* New York: Pantheon.

Howe, D. A., Chapman, N. J., & Baggett, S. A. (1994). *Planning for an aging society.* (Planning Advisory Service, Report #451). Washington, DC: American Planning Association.

Liberty, R. L. (2003). Abolishing exclusionary zoning: A natural policy alliance for environmentalists and affordable housing advocates. *Boston College Environmental Affairs Law Review, 30*(3): 581-594.

Liebig, P. S. (2001). International perspectives on housing frail elders. *Journal of Architecture and Planning Research 18*(3): 208-222.

Linsk, N., & Keigher, S. (1995). Compensation of family care for the elderly. In R. Kane and J. D. Penrod (Eds.), *Family caregiving in an aging society.* Thousand Oaks, CA: Sage.

McCamant, K., & Durret, C. (1998). *Cohousing: A contemporary approach to housing ourselves.* Berkeley, CA: Habitat Press.

National Alliance for Caregiving and AARP (1997). *Family caregiving in the U.S.: Findings from a national survey, final report.* Retrieved September 2004 from http://nac.org.

Nelson, A. C. (2003). Top ten state and local strategies to increase affordable housing supply. *Housing facts & findings, 5*(1): 1, 4-7.

Pindell, T. (1995). *A good place to live.* New York: Henry Holt.

Pollak, P. B. (1994). Rethinking zoning to accommodate the elderly in single family housing. *Journal of the American Planning Association, 60*(4), 521-539.

Pollak, P. B., & Gorman, A. N. (1989). *Community-based housing for the elderly: A zoning guide for planners and municipal officials* (Planning Advisory Service, Report # 420). Washington, DC: American Planning Association.

Pynoos, J., & Golant, S. M. (1995). Housing and living arrangements for the elderly. In R. H. Binstock and L. K. George (Eds.), *Handbook of aging and the social sciences* (4th ed.). San Diego: Academic Press.

Pynoos, J., & Liebig, P. S. (1995). Policies, trends, and implications. In J. Pynoos and P. S. Liebig (Eds.), *Housing frail elders: International policies, perspectives, and prospects.* Baltimore: Johns Hopkins University Press.

Pynoos, J., & Redfoot, D. L. (1995). Housing frail elders in the United States. In J. Pynoos and P. S. Liebig (Eds.), *Housing frail elders: International policies, perspectives, and prospects.* Baltimore: Johns Hopkins University.

Quang Do., A. (2002). Zoning. In L. A. Vitt (Ed.), *Encyclopedia of Retirement and Finance, II*, pp. 798-802. Westport, CT: Greenwood Press.

Sickle, J. M., & Kascal, J. A. (1984). Housing options: Three variations. *Journal of Housing, 41*(3): 75-77.

Uhlenberg, P. (2000). Integration of old and young. *The Gerontologist, 40*(3): 276-279.

U.S. Census Bureau (2001a). American housing survey of the United States in 2001: Historical census of housing tables, 1900-2000. (AHS/HUD Series H-150). Retrieved September, 2004 from *www.census.gov.hhes/housing/ahs/nationaldata.html*

U.S. Census Bureau (2001b). American housing survey of the United States in 2001: Household composition-Occupied units. (AHS/HUD Series H-150-29). Retrieved September, 2004 from *www.census.gov.hhes/housing/ahs/ahs01/tab29.html*

U.S. Department of Housing and Urban Development (1999). *Housing our elders: A report on housing conditions and the needs of older Americans.* Washington, DC: Author.

Wilmoth, J. M. (2001). Living arrangements among older immigrants in the United States. *The Gerontologist, 41*(2): 228-238.

doi:10.1300/J031v18n03_11

Resident and Family Perspectives on Assisted Living

Carrie A. Levin, PhD

Rutgers University

Rosalie A. Kane, DSW

University of Minnesota

SUMMARY. This research describes and compares the relative importance residents and family members place on attributes of the environment, the programs, and the policies of assisted living; describes their
satisfaction with these features; and identifies factors associated with
congruence between residents' and family members' ratings of importance and satisfaction. Both residents and their family members had high
importance and satisfaction ratings. Family members gave the assisted
living setting lower satisfaction ratings on all features than did residents.
Congruence ranged from 34% to 71% for importance items and from
29% to 63% for satisfaction. Female residents, affectionate family relationships, and residing in an AL owned by a chain were positively associated with congruence on importance items, while resident and family
education, resident income, and family involvement were negatively
associated with congruence on importance items. For congruence on
satisfaction items, having an affectionate relationship was positively associated and higher ADL dependency, more family involvement at the
facility, and family members who viewed the facility as a safe place

[Haworth co-indexing entry note]: "Resident and Family Perspectives on Assisted Living." Levin, Carrie
A., and Rosalie A. Kane. Co-published simultaneously in *Journal of Aging & Social Policy* (The Haworth
Press, Inc.) Vol. 18, No. 3/4, 2006, pp. 173-192; and: *Family and Aging Policy* (ed: Francis G. Caro) The
Haworth Press, Inc., 2006, pp. 173-192. Single or multiple copies of this article are available for a fee from
The Haworth Document Delivery Service [1-800-HAWORTH, 9:00 a.m. - 5:00 p.m. (EST). E-mail address:
docdelivery@haworthpress. com].

were negatively associated with congruence. This study makes a major stride forward because cognitively intact residents' perspectives are compared and contrasted with their own family members' perspectives, thus showing that residents and family members are two distinct groups, each with a unique set of preferences. doi:10.1300/J031v18n03_12 *[Article copies available for a fee from The Haworth Document Delivery Service: 1-800-HAWORTH. E-mail address: <docdelivery@haworthpress.com> Website: <http://www.HaworthPress.com> © 2006 by The Haworth Press, Inc. All rights reserved.]*

KEYWORDS. Assisted living, long-term care, consumer satisfaction

INTRODUCTION

Policymakers and consumer advocates are urging consumer involvement in all aspects of health care, including long-term care (LTC) (Applebaum, Straker, & Geron, 2000; GAO, 1997; GAO, 1999; Hawes, Rose, & Phillips, 1999; IOM, 2001; Pascoe & Attkisson, 1983; Ware, Davies-Avery, & Stewart, 1978). Accordingly, consumers are often included in quality assessments through the use of satisfaction surveys (Applebaum, Straker, & Geron, 2000; Smith, 2000; Donabedian, 1980). But in residentially based LTC, the identity of the consumer is ambiguous (Smith, 2000), and, in fact, providers are aware that they are serving multiple customers–the resident and the family (Applebaum et al., 2000). Because family members are often the ones who make decisions regarding admissions or are the ones paying the bills, providers may view family members as their primary customers (National Investment Conference, 1998). Therefore, it is important that providers as well as regulatory agencies be concerned with aspects of care and life within assisted living (AL) that contribute to quality from both the resident and the family perspective.

Very little research has been done examining the differences between resident and family member perceptions of care and life in LTC. Family members' preferences are often used as proxies for residents when the residents are not able to answer for themselves, but their views are not considered when residents are cognitively intact. In contrast, this study makes a major stride forward in this regard because cognitively intact residents' perspectives are compared and contrasted with their *own* family members' perspectives. The reality of decision making in LTC is that it is an interaction between residents and their family members, even though they may have different emphases and goals. Therefore, ascertaining the preferences and satisfaction of both residents and family members is important to ensure that LTC facilities can meet the needs of all consumers.

There is a dearth of published research on quality, preferences, and satisfaction in AL. This research expands upon the work done by Greene and colleagues (1997), the National Investment Conference (1998), and Gesell (2001) to provide a quantitative analysis of the preferences and perceptions of AL residents and their family members. Although studies comparing the views of older people and their family members regarding end of life decisions and various medical treatment have uncovered discrepancies(Gerety, Chiodo, Kanten, Tuley, & Cornell, 1993; Mattimore et al., 1997; Ouslander, Tymchuk, & Rahbar, 1989; Uhlmann, Pearlman, & Cain, 1988), this is one of the first studies to examine congruence between older people and their families on the very nature of residentially-based LTC. This study examines the preferences and actual evaluative judgments of 350 pairs of cognitively intact residents of AL and their close family members who live outside the AL setting. It examines these different perspectives of what constitutes quality of care and quality of life in one type of residential care facility–AL–taking into account that apartment-style AL aspires to combine high quality personal care and nursing services with a homelike and natural living environment with a philosophy that emphasizes dignity, choice, independence, privacy, and normal lifestyles for the older individual (Kane & Wilson, 1993; Mollica, 1998; Wilson, 1996).

METHODS

The Conceptual Model

The conceptual model for this research is based on Strasser and colleagues' (1993) model of satisfaction and the premise that residents and family members have different preferences and perceptions of AL based on their different goals, roles, and priorities. This model, thus, suggests that individual differences in experiences between people explain differences in value judgments and therefore, ratings of importance and satisfaction. The present study explores characteristics of individuals and their environments that may help to explain patterns in attitude, namely satisfaction formation.

Sample

The sample was drawn from six states with a substantial supply of apartment-style AL, Medicaid coverage of AL, and a variety of policies regarding what was permitted, required, or prohibited in AL, namely Arizona, Florida, Massachusetts, Minnesota, New Jersey, and Texas. Within each state, we drew a multi-county geographic area around a major urban hub. The universe included all "apartment-style" AL settings in the target counties. All settings were self-contained units with an outside door, a full bathroom, and a kitchenette with at least 10 residents that offered two meals a day in a common dining room and provided or arranged housekeeping, personal care, and routine nursing services. In each state, we chose a random sample of 10 facilities, stratified to include equally numbers of urban, rural, and larger and smaller facilities. In our sampling scheme, we also constrained the state sample so it would not contain more than two facilities of the same owner. Ten facilities in each state were chosen for a total of 60 facilities. Given the sample size, we intended no generalization back to the county, region, or states. A protracted process was needed to enumerate the eligible AL apartment-style programs. Only three eligible facilities refused to participate, and these were replaced by the next randomly selected facility within the size and geographic stratum required.

We then randomly selected 10 residents in each facility for a total of 600 residents. Eligibility included: age 65 and above, residing in the AL for at least a week at baseline, and not be terminally ill. Because our goal was to examine the congruence in preferences and perceptions of the AL facility between the resident and his or her own family member who lives outside of the facility, the comparison would not be possible if the proxy and family member were the same person, so residents who required proxy respondents to complete their interview were excluded from this study. During the resident interview, all residents were asked to identify the individual (family or friend) living outside the facility who had the greatest involvement in their lives and who had phone or in-person contact with them within the past month. These individuals constituted the family sample.

Data Collection

Residents were interviewed in-person. The resident questionnaire contained questions regarding demographic characteristics; care needs; health, mental, and functional status; psychological well-being; social functioning; service use; a scale to determine which facility attributes are important to them; a scale to measure satisfaction with various facility attributes; and global satisfaction measures. Family member data were collected by mail and questions paralleled those asked the residents. Family members were asked to respond from their own perspectives, not as proxies for the residents. A phone interview with each facility's administrator was used to obtain information about facility size, occupancy rate, how long it has been in business, whether it accepts Medicaid, location, types of services, staffing, cost for services, and rent. Additionally, a baseline resident phone audit was conducted to gather information about each resident's functioning, services, cost for services, and rent.

Measures

Measures used in the analyses are described in Table 1. The two dependent variables, importance ratings and satisfaction ratings, are summarized below. Also described is a measure of family members' perceptions of their relationships with the residents and affectional integration, which was adapted from the work of Bengtson (Mangen, Bengtson et al., 1988).

Importance Ratings. Likert-type items were used to measure the importance ratings of facility attributes that may or may not be important to the residents and their family members. Attributes were chosen based on a review of the literature relevant to the measurement of resident satisfaction and the quality of care for individuals residing in AL including: convenience of apartment; comfort and attractiveness of apartment; kitchen appliances; privacy; quality of menus and meals in dining room; atmosphere and service in dining room; housekeeping; laundry; personal care assistance; nursing consultation; nighttime assistance; medication assistance; regularity of staffing; activities; physical rehabilitation; transportation; religious services/programs; ability to decorate and arrange apartment; decisions regarding amount of assistance; decisions regarding who enters apartment and when; ability to refuse recommended services; aging in place; having things in common with other residents. First, a stem question was asked:

TABLE 1. Measures Used for Comparison of Resident and Family Perspective

VARIABLE NAME	SOURCE	MEASUREMENT
Congruence Importance OLS	Resident Questionnaire Family Questionnaire	Continuous (0-23): count of congruent importance questions for each resident/family dyad
Congruence Satisfaction OLS	Resident Questionnaire Family Questionnaire	Continuous (0-23): count of congruent satisfaction questions for each resident/family dyad
Resident Age	Resident Questionnaire	Continuous: number of years of age
Resident Gender	Baseline Resident Audit	Dichotomous: 0 = male, 1 = female
Resident Education	Resident Questionnaire	Dichotomous:0 = less than high school graduate, 1 = completed high school +
Resident Income	Resident Questionnaire	Dichotomous: 0 = $20,000 +, 1 = < $20,000 annually
Length of Stay (LOS)	Baseline Resident Audit	Continuous: number of months resident has lived at AL
Self Perceived Health	Resident Questionnaire	Dichotomous: 0 = good to excellent, 1 = fair to poor
Mental Status (MSQ) (Pfeiffer, 1975)	Resident Questionnaire	Dichotomous: 0 = 3 or fewer MSQ errors, 1 = > 3 MSQ errors
Psychological Well-being (Ware & Sherbourne, 1992)	Resident Questionnaire	Continuous: Scale ranging from 0-100 with a high score indicating high psychological well-being.
Chronic Illness	Resident Questionnaire	Continuous (0-6): Sum of chronic illnesses including: COPD; CHF; Cancer; Parkinson's; Stroke within the past year; MS
Assistive Device	Resident Questionnaire	Continuous (0-6): Sum of assistive devices used: cane; walker; wheelchair; electric cart; continence products; mechanical lift
Hospital	Resident Questionnaire	Dichotomous: 0 = has not been hospitalized in past 6 months, 1 = has been hospitalized
ADL sum	Resident Questionnaire	Continuous (0-6): Sum of ADL assistance with high score indicating greater dependence in bathing; dressing; transferring; eating; toileting; getting around indoors.
IADL sum	Resident Questionnaire	Continuous (0-8): Sum of IADL assistance with high score indicating greater dependence in medication; housekeeping; laundry; shopping; driving medical; driving social; managing finances; making appointments.
Unmet needs (Allen & Mor, 1997)	Resident Questionnaire	Continuous (0-13), number of unmet ADL and IADL care needs
Outside activities	Resident Questionnaire	Dichotomous: 0 = participated in outside activities less than weekly, 1 = participated in outside activities about weekly or more
Good conversation	Resident Questionnaire	Dichotomous: 0 = less than daily good conversations with other residents, 1 = daily conversation with other residents
Organized activities	Resident Questionnaire	Dichotomous: 0 = participated in organized activities less than weekly, 1 = participated in organized activities about weekly or more
Solo activities	Resident Questionnaire	Dichotomous: 0 = does solo activities less than daily 1 = does solo activities daily
Child of resident	Family Questionnaire	Dichotomous: 0 = not child, 1 = son or daughter
Family Education	Family Questionnaire	Dichotomous: 0 = less than college degree, 1 = college degree
Family Gender	Family Questionnaire	Dichotomous: 0 = male, 1 = female
Family Involvement	Family Questionnaire	Combination of care assistance and contact: 0 = visited less than weekly and did not provide more than 3.5 hours of assistance, 1 = visited about weekly or more and provide 3.5 or more hours of assistance
Affectional Integration (Mangen, Bengtson et al. 1988)	Family Questionnaire	Continuous: Scale from 5-30 with higher scores indicating high affection between resident and family member
Family pays for services or rent	Family Questionnaire	Dichotomous: 0 = no financial assistance from family respondent, 1 = study participant contributes financially to resident
Safe	Family Questionnaire	Dichotomous: 0 = family rates facility very safe, 1 = family rates facility as less than very safe
Facility Size	Administrative Interview	Dichotomous: 0 = less than 60 units, 1 = 60 or more units
Facility part of a chain	Administrative Interview	Dichotomous: 0 = not owned by an AL chain, 1 = owned by a chain
Medicaid	Administrative Interview	Dichotomous: 0 = does not have any Medicaid residents, 1 = has Medicaid residents
Rural	Rural Urban Continuum Code	Dichotomous: 0 = metropolitan area, 1 = rural

We'd like to know what's important to you in a place to live and get services. I will go through a list of things that may or may not be important to you and ask you to rate the importance of each as 1, 2, 3, 4, or 5. "1" means the lowest importance and "5" means the highest. This is not about [NAME OF FACILITY] but just about what you generally think is important, whether [NAME OF FACILITY] has it or not. How important to you is [INTERVIEWERS, FILL IN SPECIFIC ITEM]:

Then respondents rated each of 23 facility characteristics for how important they believed each was for them to have that particular attribute in a place where they live and receive care.

Satisfaction Ratings. Identical Likert-type items to those items used to rate importance were used to measure satisfaction ratings for each facility attribute. Respondents were asked:

Now I would like you to give me your confidential rating of [FACILITY NAME] on a number of features. Please rate [FACILITY NAME] with 1, 2, 3, 4, or 5 with 1 being the lowest possible score and 5 the highest. We'd like your ratings even on things that are not especially important to you. Taking it all together, how would you score [FACILITY NAME] on [INTERVIEWERS FILL IN SPECIFIC ITEMS]:

The family questionnaire was designed specifically for use in answering the research questions for this study. Many of the questions mirror questions in the resident questionnaire so that direct comparisons could be made, including a parallel form of the importance and satisfaction questions. The remaining questions elicited information from family members about their backgrounds, demographic characteristics, and their relationships with relatives in the AL, including care they provide.

Affectional Integration. Because the purpose of the parent study (resident survey) was to examine patterns of care in AL, no measure representing the relationship between the resident and her or his family member was included. In the present study, we added a measure of the family member's perception of the affectional relationship between him or her and the resident, as a possible variable affecting congruence. Affection between a family member and his or her relative was measured using the affectional solidarity scale created for the University of Southern California Longitudinal Study of Generations (Mangen et al., 1988). This scale consists of five items: (1) present closeness of relationship;

(2) communication; (3) how well respondent and relative get along together; (4) how well respondent understands relative; and (5) how well respondent feels relative understands him or her. Individual items are summed to create a scale of family affection that ranges from 5 (low affection) to 30 (high affection) (Gronvold, 1988).

Analytic Techniques

Principal components factor analysis was conducted to determine the factor structure of both the 23 importance and 23 satisfaction rating items in order to reduce the data into domains. Using a conservative guideline, factor loadings greater than or equal to .50 were used and those less than .50 were dropped (Comrey & Lee, 1992). It was determined a priori that if discrepancies emerged, the factors resulting from the residents would be used because they are the primary consumers of AL. The reliability of each domain sub-scale was tested. A group mean level of importance was created for each domain separately for residents as a group and family members as a group by summing the mean importance rating on each attribute within the domain. Independent samples t-tests with Bonferroni corrections (Tukey, 1991) were performed to compare means in each domain between residents and family members.

Realistically, we did not expect residents and their family members to demonstrate exact correspondence between their responses although responses were skewed highly towards the positive for both importance and satisfaction ratings. Therefore, residents' and family members' response categories for each individual importance and satisfaction item were collapsed from five (1, 2, 3, 4, 5) to three (1-3, 4, 5) before calculating congruence for a particular item. For example, for the satisfaction item regarding having a comfortable and attractive apartment, suppose the resident gave a response of 3 and her daughter gave a 2. Using the collapsed categories, this dyad received a 1, representing congruence, for this item.

Congruence item $X_i = 1$ if resident and family member give same responses

Congruence item $X_i = 0$ if resident and family member give different responses

Two analyses have been done to examine congruence between resident/family member dyads. First, congruence between each resident and his or her own family member was calculated for each facility characteristic and then summed across variables to create two summary dependent variables: congruence$_{importance}$ and congruence$_{satisfaction}$:

congruence$_{important}$ = Σ (X$_i$)
congruence$_{satisfaction}$ = Σ (X$_i$)

Estimation was done using ordinary least squares regression.

$$Y = \beta 0 + \beta_i Z_i + \gamma$$

Where Y = congruence$_{importance/satisfaction}$
Z$_i$ = explanatory variables (resident, family, facility characteristics).

Explanatory variables included in each model are listed in Table 1.

RESULTS

Sample

Responses from family members and residents were used in this analysis only when we had a response from both the resident and family member. One hundred and eight residents were not eligible because either they: had no family (N = 21), refused to provide a family contact (N = 35), listed another resident in the AL (N = 2), provided the name of someone who was not a family member (e.g., paid professionals) (N = 8), had a proxy (N = 39), or were under age 65 (N = 2). This left 492 residents whose family members were eligible to participate in this study. From this 492, additional exclusions included family members of residents who died (N = 6) or relocated (N = 15) before addresses were obtained, and survey questionnaires that were returned undeliverable (N = 12). This left a possible universe of 459 dyads whom we located and for whom we might have had responses. One hundred and nine did not complete questionnaires, including 101 who did not reply; four who replied and refused to complete the survey; three replied that the resident was deceased and did not complete the survey; and one who could not complete due to health problems, leaving a sample of 350 resident/family member dyads used in the final analyses. Although no incentives were used, a 76.3% response rate was achieved from those family members using an initial mailing, a reminder postcard, and two follow-up mailings.

The resident and family member sample characteristics did not differ by state. Profiles of residents and family members are similar to samples reported in other national AL studies (Mollica, 1998; Hawes et al., 1999). The sample of residents was predominately female, with a mean age of 86, and a mean length of stay of 22 months. The family sample was predominately female with a mean age of 59 years, and provided a median of 3.5 hours of care assistance (not including visiting) for their relatives each week. Detailed demographic information is available from the lead author upon request.

Factor Analysis

Exploratory factor analysis of the residents' importance items suggests the presence of five factors among residents. After dropping items that loaded with less than .5 or that were not discriminant in loading on just one factor, a clean factor analysis resulted with five factors: Control and Choice; Household; Care; Programs; and Dining. For satisfaction items, results suggest the presence of six factors: Programs; Control and Choice; Care; Dining; Household Services; and Living Situation. Contact lead author for complete factor analyses results.

The reliability of each domain sub-scale was tested. All reliabilities fell within the acceptable range (Nunnally & Bernstein, 1994). The all-item scale reliability was .86 for residents and .85 for families. The Cronbach's alpha for each of the five importance domains: household (resident (res) α = .72, family (fam) α = .66); control and choice (res α = .78, fam α = .70); care (res α = .73 fam α = .61); programs (res α = .73, fam α = .71); and dining (res α = .73, fam α = .81). The Cronbach's alpha for each of the six satisfaction domains: living situation (res α = .48, fam α = .57); household services (res α = .71, fam α = .73); control and choice (res α = .62, fam α = .70); care (res α = .71, fam α = .80); programs (res α = .70, fam α = .75); and dining (res α = .73, fam α = .82). Using the decision criteria to drop items that did not load with at least .5 on a factor and with greater than a .20 spread between loadings, many of the family members' items were dropped from the factor analysis. Taking this into consideration, the factor structures of the residents and family members did not differ significantly; therefore, we found that the alpha reliabilities for family members were higher than residents for the satisfaction domains, which is most likely due to the fact that items that did not have a large distribution of values were dropped from the factor analyses.

Mean Importance and Satisfaction Ratings

There were no significant differences between residents' and family members' composite ratings of importance in the dining domain or the household domain. Family members' composite importance ratings were significantly higher than residents' composite importance ratings for the control and choice, care and programs domains. There were no significant differences between residents' and family members' composite ratings of satisfaction in the living situation domain. Family members did not have any composite satisfaction ratings that were higher than the residents. See Tables 2 and 3 for complete comparisons.

Congruence

Table 4 presents the rates of congruence from the individual importance and satisfaction items. For the importance items, congruence ranged from a low of 33.6% for having the same people help you regularly to a high of 70.7% for having someone on duty in the building at night. For the satisfaction items, congruence ranged from a low of 28.8% for having laundry done the way you like to a high of 63.1% for being able to decorate and arrange how you want.

TABLE 2. Comparisons of Residents' and Family Members' Importance Ratings by Domain

		Residents (N = 350)		Family Members (N = 350)		
	Domain (possible score)	Mean	(SD)	Mean	(SD)	t
IMPORTANCE RATINGS	Control (4-20)	14.97	(4.82)	16.76	(2.83)	5.99**
	Household (4-20)	17.81	(2.68)	17.76	(2.16)	-.27
	Care (4-20)	16.85	(3.88)	18.02	(2.51)	4.74**
	Programs (4-20)	14.29	(4.36)	15.78	(3.33)	5.07**
	Dining (2-10)	9.27	(1.35)	9.46	(1.05)	2.06

**Bonferroni corrected p < .01

TABLE 3. Comparisons of Residents' and Family Members' Satisfaction Ratings by Domain

		Residents (N = 350)		Family Members (N = 350)		
Domain (possible score)		Mean	(SD)	Mean	(SD)	t
SATISFACTION RATINGS	Control (4-20)	17.59	(2.07)	16.74	(2.58)	−4.75**
	Household Services (2-10)	8.73	(1.50)	7.29	(1.84)	−11.30**
	Care (4-20)	17.91	(2.33)	15.81	(3.44)	−9.43**
	Programs (4-20)	14.87	(3.17)	13.45	(3.77)	−5.35**
	Dining (2-10)	8.33	(1.73)	7.57	(2.10)	−5.26**
	Living Situation (2-10)	8.63	(1.62)	8.48	(1.68)	−1.25

**Bonferroni corrected p < .01

TABLE 4. Congruence and Non-Congruence Among Assisted Living Residents and Their Family Members: Importance & Rating Items

Item	Importance Congruence (percent)	Rating Congruence (percent)
Having the same people help you regularly	33.6	30.8
Having organized activities for the residents	35.6	33.7
Being able to refuse recommended services	37.6	38.3
Having things in common with other residents	38.5	36.9
Deciding how much or little care or help you receive	40.5	37.2
Being allowed to age in place	41.1	30.3
Having physical rehabilitation programs like PT	41.9	58.8
Deciding who comes into your apartment and when	43.7	47.5
Having transportation arranged for the building	45.4	33.4
Having a refrigerator and stove/microwave in apartment	46.3	39.5
Being able to decorate and arrange how you want	46.8	63.1
Having religious services & programs in building	47.1	36.3
Having laundry done the way you like	47.7	28.8
Having an apt. designed for people with disabilities	49.7	40.6
Having housekeeping done the way you like	50.0	31.4
Being able to lock your apartment door for privacy	55.5	53.9
Having a nurse in the building	59.2	36.3
Having a comfortable and attractive apartment	60.1	52.7
Having help available for taking medicines	60.3	44.4
Having assistance available for personal care	60.3	35.4
Having meals that you like in the dining room	61.5	42.9
Having pleasant service & atmosphere in dining room	65.2	44.4
Having someone on duty in the building at night	70.7	40.1

Predictors of Overall Congruence

The results of the robust OLS regression for congruence between family member/resident dyads on importance items are summarized in Table 5. The model accounts for 15% of the variance (adjusted R^2) in congruence on importance ratings. The results show that congruence is influenced by a positive affectional relationship between resident and family member. Additionally, residents and family members have a higher congruence score if the resident resides in a facility owned by an AL chain. Resident gender (being female) and income are positively re-

TABLE 5. OLS Estimates of Congruence Between Residents' and Family Members' Importance and Satisfaction Ratings Coefficients and Standard Errors

Predictor	Importance Congruence	SE	P value	Satisfaction Congruence	SE	P value
Resident age			ns			ns
Resident gender (1 = female)	1.238	(.537)	p = .025			ns
Resident education (1 = high school +)	−.899	(.444)	p =.047			ns
Resident income (1 = < $20,000 annually)	−1.195	(.520)	p =.025			ns
Resident length of stay			ns			ns
Resident self-reported health (1 = fair to poor)			ns			ns
Resident mental status (1 = 3+ mistakes)			ns			ns
Resident psychological well-being			ns			ns
# of chronic illnesses (resident)			ns			ns
# of assistive devices (resident)			ns			ns
Hospital (1 = hospitalized within last 6 mo.)			ns			ns
ADL sum (res.)			ns	−.580	(.181)	p =.002
IADL sum (res.)			ns			ns
# of unmet ADL and IADL needs (resident)			ns			ns
Res. participates in outside activities (1 = weekly +)			ns			ns
Res. has daily good conversations (1 = daily+)			ns			ns
Res. participates in activities (1 = weekly +)			ns			ns
Res. participates in solo activities (1 = daily +)			ns			ns
Child of resident (1 = son/daughter)			ns			ns
Family education (1 = college +)	−1.250	(.391)	p =.002			ns
Family gender (1 = female)			ns			ns
High family involvement (1 = high involvement)	−.972	(.483)	p =.049	−.913	(.417)	p =.032
Affectional integration	.119	(.052)	p =.025	.126	(.046)	p =.008
Family pays for services (1 = family pays)			ns			ns
Family feels AL is safe (1 = unsafe)			ns	−.754	(.370)	p =.045
Facility size (1 = 60+ units)			ns			ns
Facility owned by a chain (1 = chain owned)	1.158	(.527)	p =.032			ns
Facility has residents on Medicaid (1 = yes)			ns			ns
Facility rural (1 = rural)			ns			ns

lated to congruence, while education is negatively related. Family education however, has a negative relationship to congruence. The more education family members have, the lower the congruence score. A resident's social functioning does not appear significantly to influence whether or not there will be congruence between the resident and the family member on importance items. Finally, the type of relationship between family member and resident (e.g., parent/child is not an important predictor of congruence, but the amount of involvement, defined as spending time with as well as providing assistance to the resident) is a predictor of congruence. The more involved a family member is in the resident's life, the lower the congruence score on importance items.

The results of the robust OLS regression of congruence between family member/resident dyads on satisfaction items are also summarized in Table 5. The model accounts for 16% of the variance in congruence on satisfaction ratings, which is quite a high explanatory power for a satisfaction study. The results imply that the more functional impairment (ADLs) a resident has, the less congruence there is on satisfaction items. Two characteristics of the relationship between residents and family members influence congruence. Family members who were more involved in residents' lives through visits and assistance were associated with lower congruence scores. The family member's rating of safety at the facility was positively related to congruence. If the family member believed the facility to be a very safe place for his or her relative to live, there is a positive association with congruence scores on satisfaction items. No other significant associations were found.

DISCUSSION

We hypothesized that residents' ratings of importance on amenities of the facility as well as features that allow them to have greater choice and control would be higher than their family members' importance ratings on these features. In addition, we hypothesized that family members would rate care provision and the availability of care and programs higher than residents. The results indicate that family members rated items in the control and choice domain higher and suggest that family members are more interested in making sure that their relatives reside in a community that offers a variety of care and programs so that the facility is able to meet their care needs. These findings support our initial hypothesis that family members are concerned with their relatives' safety and care. Perhaps this is because residents know their abilities and limitations and therefore rate facility features thinking only of their present situations, whereas family members may feel that facilities ought to offer a wide variety of care, programs, and services to meet any need that may arise.

We hypothesized that residents would be more critical of features of the facility because they have more experience with them than their family members. Family members may not have ever tasted the food in the dining room or joined in any activities. A family member may know that a variety of activities is offered daily and give a high rating for activities, whereas a resident knows that there are a number of activities offered, but does not care for the selection. Our data indicate just the opposite; residents had higher satisfaction ratings on all satisfaction domains where a statistically significant difference between residents and family members exists. Perhaps this is due to the fact that residents may be more influenced by personal characteristics of their providers and the facility staff, such as their interpersonal skills or the environment in which the care is provided, in making judgments, rather than basing their assessments on the quality of the services provided. An alternative explanation is that older consumers, especially consumers of LTC, are dependent on their providers for meeting basic daily living requirements and therefore may be reluctant to disclose any negative ratings of their care for fear of retribution. Another possibility is that residents are giving higher ratings because to them, being in an AL is a much more satisfying alternative compared to being in a nursing home. It is as good as can be expected for individuals who do not live independently. Higher satisfaction ratings may also represent a cohort effect. This generation of older adults might be less likely to criticize their providers and setting than their relatives.

Because we asked family members to respond from their own perspectives rather than as proxies for their relatives, we expected their responses to differ from residents because of their unique set of expectations and perceptions of AL. Yet, there was a great deal of congruence between residents and their family members. On individual importance items, both groups responded similarly regarding having assistance available (personal care, medicine, at night) as well as having food that the resident likes served in the dining room. For satisfaction items, residents and family members tended to be congruent in response on items dealing with allowing the resident's personal environment (decorating the apartment the way the resident chooses and having a comfortable apartment).

Limitations

The sample of facilities within each state was purposeful rather than a random selection. Therefore, results cannot be generalized to AL facilities nationwide. We may have sample selection bias; those facilities willing to participate in the study may differ significantly from those not willing to participate. Therefore, the results are only generalizable to residents sharing similar characteristics living in facilities with characteristics similar to those participating in this study. There is also potential for positive response bias from family members. Family members willing to return the questionnaire may differ from those who chose not to answer the questionnaire. Respondents are probably relatives who have better relationships and more contact with the residents than those who did not choose to complete the questionnaire. Finally, because this family study was appended to an existing study, we were limited to the available resident data and were unable to collect data from residents about their perceptions of the affectional relationship with family members.

Future Research

Future research might examine importance, satisfaction, and congruence as independent variables. Specifically: (1) Are importance ratings, satisfaction ratings, and/or congruence linked to the family members and residents giving referrals to others who are interested in entering an AL? (2) Are importance, satisfaction, and congruence scores linked to relocation and if so, do they lead to relocation to another facility serving a similar population; do they make a lateral move; or do they move to a different type of facility that serves a different level of acuity? (3) Is congruence linked to familial problems in the future?

A second area of future research might focus on longitudinal analyses. Specifically, does what's important to individuals change over time? Greene and colleagues (1997) found that family members' perceptions of what was important changed over time. Additionally, it is important to examine whether satisfaction and congruence change over time. Perceptions and importance ratings are value assessments, and as such, we need to examine the extent to which the kinds of values and preferences that are reported are stable over time. An ideal study would include studying perspectives of residents and family members before the resident entered the facility, including what their expectations were; during their experience in the AL; and after they leave the facility.

It would be interesting to extend the study to include more than one family member for each resident to see how the perspectives between family and resident differ and to examine the difference in perspective between various family members. We would gain a great deal of understanding about families if we conduct a more comprehensive study of the family relationship including information regarding the relationship between family members and residents throughout the life course of the resident, including the time immediately prior to entering the AL.

Further exploration into understanding the meaning of discrepancies in perspectives between residents and family members is necessary. When, if ever, do we want to see concordance? Under what circumstances do we want to have congruence? When is it good to have congruence and when is it not good? Why do residents and family members evaluate or value similar characteristics of the facility in different ways? Do disparities exist because of the nature of facility characteristics? Are residents and family members more likely to be in concordance on facts and less likely to concur on items that deal with beliefs? Is there a pattern that can be teased out to describe disparities? These are all questions that need further attention.

POLICY IMPLICATIONS

We have shown that there are indeed two separate markets of consumers in AL: residents and their family members. Now, it must be determined which consumer is sovereign and which is secondary. In essence, family members cannot be used as proxies. They do indeed have different perspectives regarding the living situation, care, and services in ALs. This has important policy implications. Up until now, we have often used family members as proxies for long-term care residents. Now that we know that they are two separate consumers with two separate sets of wants and needs, we should not use family as proxies for resident respondents if it is possible to interview a resident directly. This has direct implications both for internal quality measurement within facilities and more broadly for public reporting of information as well as regulatory policies.

There is a move toward public reporting of consumer feedback across the health care industry. In managed care, consumers provide feedback via report cards and many states are beginning to or planning to collect and publicly report LTC satisfaction information (Lowe, Lucas, Castle, Robinson, & Crystal, 2003). Quality of care and service are major concerns for all consumers, providers, and regulators of AL services. This study shows that in order to provide a complete picture of AL, it is necessary to report satisfaction results from both residents and family members. The results of this study are useful in allowing facilities to understand and focus on what residents and their families value in a place to live and receive assistance. The recent growth in the quality assurance industry focuses on consumer preferences. The assessments made by residents and their family members are representative of a way to measure consumer choice in the selection of an AL residence. For satisfaction results to be useful, providers must be willing to conduct ongoing surveys of what is important to their consumers and then see how they are doing in terms of providing for their wants and needs. It is necessary for providers to go the next step, not just to collect information on preferences, but to act on them. Providers need to hear what consumers are telling them and act upon their advice. Additionally, regulatory agencies should consider making satisfaction information available from both residents and family members.

Findings from this study suggest that it is important to honor and respect resident and family member preferences for various aspects of their living situation and care. Resources need to be allocated to ensure that we place value on respecting these preferences–there is a push toward more regulation of AL, and this study provides evidence that both residents and family members value a living situation that supports residents' needs while allowing for individual choice. Currently, AL is a LTC option that offers more choice and control than a nursing home, but it is an industry that is becoming more regulated with many regulations centering on restricting customer-centered care to protect resident health and safety. It is possible that consumers may want to assume risk in order to maximize benefits other than those of health or safety to enrich their quality of life. Our findings show that features of the AL facilities other than those solely regarding care are important to residents and their family members and thus, features that support and improve quality of life need to be considered in provider planning as well as in regulation of AL.

AUTHOR NOTES

Dr. Levin is Assistant Research Professor at the Institute for Health, Health Policy, and Aging Research at Rutgers University. She can be contacted at IHHCPAR, Rutgers University, 30 College Avenue, New Brunswick, NJ 08901 (E-mail: clevin@ihhcpar. rutgers.edu).

Dr. Kane is Professor in the Division of Health Services Research and Policy at the School of Public Health at the University of Minnesota.

This study was partly funded by the Robert Wood Johnson Foundation through its funding of a study called The Assisted Living/Home Care Research Initiative, as part of the Home Care Research Initiative, administered by the Visiting Nurse Service of New York City.

REFERENCES

Allen, S. M., & Mor, V. (1997). The prevalence and consequences of unmet need. Contrasts between older and younger adults with disability. *Medical Care, 35*(11): 1132-1148.

Applebaum, R. A., Straker, J. K., & Geron, S. M. (2000). *Assessing satisfaction in health and long-term care.* New York: Springer Publishing Company, Inc.

Comrey, A. L., & Lee, H. B. (1992). *A first course in factor analysis* (2nd ed.). Hillsdale, NJ: Erlbaum.

Donabedian, A. (1980). *Explorations in quality assessment and monitoring: The definition of quality and approaches to its assessment.* (Vol. 1). Ann Arbor, MI: Health Administration Press.

GAO (1997). *Long-term care: Consumer protection and quality-of-care issues in assisted living.* (GAO/HEHS-97-93). Washington DC: Government Printing Office.

GAO (1999). *Assisted Living: Quality-of-care and consumer protection issues in four states.* (GAO/HEHS-99-27). Washington, DC: Government Printing Office.

Gerety, M. B., Chiodo, L. K., Kanten, D. N., Tuley, M. R., & Cornell, J. E. (1993). Medical treatment preferences of nursing home residents: Relationship to function and concordance with surrogate decision-makers. *JAGS, 41*: 953-960.

Gesell, S. B. (2001). A measure of satisfaction for the assisted-living industry. *Journal for Healthcare Quality, 23*(2): 16-25.

Greene, A., Hawes, C., Wood, M., & Woodsong, C. (1997). How do family members define quality in assisted living facilities? *Generations*, 34-36.

Gronvold, R. L. (1988). Measuring Affectual Solidarity. In D. J. Mangen, V. L. Bengtson, & P. H. Landry, Jr. (Eds.), *Measurement of Intergenerational Relations* (pp. 74-98). Newbury Park, CA: Sage Publications.

Hawes, C., Rose, M., & Phillips, C. D. (1999). *A national study of assisted living for the frail elderly.* Washington, DC: Office of Disability, Aging, and Long-Term Care. Office of the Assistant Secretary for Planning and Evaluation. U.S. Department of Health and Human Services.

Institute of Medicine (IOM) (2001). *Improving the quality of long-term care.* Washington, DC: National Academy Press.

Kane, R. A., & Wilson, K. B. (1993). *Assisted living in the United States: A new paradigm for residential care for frail elderly persons?* Washington, DC: American Association of Retired Persons

Lowe, T. J., Lucas, J. A., Castle, N. G., Robinson, J. P., & Crystal, S. (2003). Consumer satisfaction in long-term care: State initiatives in nursing homes and assisted living facilities. *The Gerontologist, 43*(6): 883-896.

Mangen, D. J., Bengtson, V. L., & Landry, P. H., Jr. (1988). *Measurement of Intergenerational Relations.* Newbury Park, CA: Sage Publications.

Mattimore, T. J., Wenger, N. S., Desbiens, N. A., Teno, J. M., Hamel, M. B., Liu, H., Califf, R., Connors, A. F., Lynn, J., & Oye, R. K. (1997). Surrogate and physician understanding of patients' preferences for living permanently in a nursing home. *JAGS, 45*: 818-824.

Mollica, R. L. (1998). *State Assisted Living Policy: 1998*. Portland, ME: National Academy for State Health Policy.

National Investment Conference (1998). *National survey of assisted living residents: Who is the consumer?* Annapolis, MD: National Investment Conference for the Senior Living and Long Term Care Industries.

Nunnally, J. C., & Bernstein, I. H. (1994). *Psychometric Theory*. (third ed.). New York, NY: McGraw-Hill, Inc.

Ouslander, J. G., Tymchuk, A. J., & Rahbar, B. (1989). Health care decision among elderly long-term care residents and their potential proxies. *Archives of Internal Medicine, 149*: 1367-1372.

Pascoe, G. C., & Attkisson, C. C. (1983). The evaluation ranking scale: A new methodology for assessing satisfaction. *Evaluation and Program Planning, 6*: 335-347.

Pfeiffer, E. (1975). A short portable mental status questionnaire for the assessment of organic brain deficit in elderly patients. *Journal of the American Geriatrics Society, 23*: 433-441.

Smith, M. (2000). Satisfaction with health and social services. In R.A. Kane, & R.A. Kane (Eds.), *Assessing the Elderly*. New York, NY: Oxford University Press.

Strasser, S., Aharony, L., & Greenberger, D. (1993). The patient satisfaction process: Moving toward a comprehensive model. *Medical Care Review, 50*(2): 219-248.

Tukey, J. W. (1991). The philosophy of multiple comparisons. *Statistical Science, 6*: 100-116.

Uhlmann, R. F., Pearlman, R. A., & Cain, K. C. (1988). Physicians' and spouses' predictions of elderly patients' resuscitation preferences. *Journal of Gerontology: Medical Sciences, 43*(5): M115-121.

Ware, J. E., Fr., Davies-Avery, A., & Stewart, A. L. (1978). The measurement and meaning of patient satisfaction. *Health and Medical Care Services Review, 1*(1): 3-15.

Ware, J. E., Jr., & Sherbourne, C. D. (1992). The MOS 36-item short-form health survey (SF-36): Conceptual framework and item selection. *Medical Care, 30*(6): 473-483.

Wilson, K. B. (1996). *Assisted living: Reconceptualizing regulation to meet consumers' needs & preferences*. Washington, DC: The American Association of Retired Persons.

doi:10.1300/J031v18n03_12

Welfare Reform:
Challenges for Grandparents
Raising Grandchildren

Casey E. Copen, MPH

University of Southern California

SUMMARY. This paper examines the impact of Temporary Aid to Needy Families (TANF) on a growing constituency that may require welfare assistance: grandparents raising grandchildren. A brief review of the demographics of grandparent caregivers is followed by an exploration of welfare reform legislation, including work requirements and the Healthy Marriage Initiative (HMI). The importance of state-level policies in assisting grandparent-headed households, particularly health care, school enrollment, and housing policies, are also discussed. The paper concludes by offering implications for welfare policies in terms of their impact on intergenerational households headed by grandparents. doi:10.1300/J031v18n03_13 *[Article copies available for a fee from The Haworth Document Delivery Service: 1-800-HAWORTH. E-mail address: <docdelivery@haworthpress.com> Website: <http://www.HaworthPress.com> © 2006 by The Haworth Press, Inc. All rights reserved.]*

KEYWORDS. Grandparents raising grandchildren, custodial grandparenting, welfare, Temporary Aid to Needy Families, federal welfare reform

[Haworth co-indexing entry note]: "Welfare Reform: Challenges for Grandparents Raising Grandchildren." Copen, Casey E.. Co-published simultaneously in *Journal of Aging & Social Policy* (The Haworth Press, Inc.) Vol. 18, No. 3/4, 2006, pp. 193-209; and: *Family and Aging Policy* (ed: Francis G. Caro) The Haworth Press, Inc., 2006, pp. 193-209. Single or multiple copies of this article are available for a fee from The Haworth Document Delivery Service [1-800-HAWORTH, 9:00 a.m. - 5:00 p.m. (EST). E-mail address: docdelivery@haworthpress. com].

Available online at http://jasp.haworthpress.com
doi:10.1300/J031v18n03_13

INTRODUCTION

The Personal Responsibility and Work Opportunity Reconciliation Act (PWORA), signed by former President Clinton in 1996, repealed Aid to Families with Dependent Children (AFDC) in favor of a block grant known as Temporary Aid to Needy Families (TANF). The transformation from AFDC, a welfare entitlement program, to TANF, an annual $16.9 billion dollar block grant, represents a monumental change in welfare's 61-year history. However, debate concerning the most efficient way to fund and administer TANF programs at the federal level continues unabated in Congress between the House of Representatives and the Senate. Despite the marked disagreement across party lines concerning the appropriation of federal welfare funds, both Democrats and Republicans have neglected to examine how the proposed changes to TANF may affect a growing constituency that may require welfare assistance: grandparents raising grandchildren.

This article contributes to past studies of TANF policy and grandparent caregivers (Mullen & Einhorn, 2000; Minkler, Berrick, & Needell, 1999) by examining the impact of TANF on grandparents who take on the role of primary caregiver for a dependent child. After a discussion of federal work requirements and the Healthy Marriage Initiative (HMI), this article explores what can be done at the state and federal levels to ensure that grandparent caregivers, and the children in their care, receive necessary assistance. The importance of state-level policies in assisting grandparent-headed households with issues such as health care, school enrollment, and housing will also be discussed. This article concludes by recommending changes to current welfare policy that would benefit grandparent caregivers and their grandchildren.

GRANDPARENTS RAISING GRANDCHILDREN: THE "SILENT SAVIORS"

The structure of American families is increasingly becoming more diverse, due to rising divorce rates, the growing number of children living in single-parent households, and the increasing longevity of older adults (Casper & Bianchi, 2002; Bengtson, 2001). The role of grandparents has become more salient in recent years as a result of these demographic and socio-historical changes. For example, longer years of "shared lives" across generations give grandparents the opportunity to provide emotional and instrumental support to children (Silverstein, Giarrusso, &

Bengtson, 1998). Similarly, grandparents play an essential role in sharing traditions, stories, and experiences with their grandchildren (King & Elder, 1999). Grandparents also provide important resources for children in times of family stress, such as parental divorce (Casper & Bianchi, 2002). Grandparents who assume the role of primary caregiver for their grandchildren are particularly influential for their grandchild's psychological well-being, as well as the child's healthy development into adulthood (Fuller-Thompson & Minkler, 2001).

The 2000 Census was the first time that questions were asked about grandparent caregivers. These questions revealed that 2.4 million grandparents were solely responsible for the basic needs of a co-residing grandchild (Simmons & Dye, 2003). In the same year, 4.4 million children were living in grandparent-headed households (Lugalia & Overturf, 2004). The most significant increase in grandparent-headed households has occurred among "skipped generation" households with no parents present, rising over 50% between 1990 and 2005 (U.S. Census Bureau, 2005). Over 1.5 million children were living with their grandparents only in 2004 (U.S. Census Bureau, 2005). African-American and Latino grandparents have an increased likelihood of taking on an extensive caregiving role, primarily because of differing family composition and unique role expectations regarding grandparenting (Goodman & Silverstein, 2002).

The number of grandparent-headed households has remained relatively stable in recent years (U.S. Census Bureau, 2005). However, there are several ways to account for the rise in grandparent caregivers, which has doubled since the 1970s. Changes in child welfare policies are one reason the number of grandparent-headed households has increased so rapidly. Today, child welfare agencies increasingly rely on relatives and other kin to care for children whose parents are absent, unable, or unwilling to provide assistance. The rise in grandparent-headed households can also be attributed to abandonment, death of the child's parent, divorce, HIV/AIDS, incarceration, mental and physical illnesses, parental drug abuse, teenage pregnancy, and unemployment.

Grandparent caregivers are most likely to take on full-time parenting roles when there are serious problems experienced by the parents, such as mental health problems, drug abuse, and incarceration (Minkler & Roe, 1996). Many grandparents describe the surrogate parenting role as a necessary, but stressful and unexpected, life transition (Cherlin & Furstenberg, 1986). One grandmother expresses the complexity and ambiguity surrounding the parenting role: "If I do too much, I have to do it all. If I do too little, I might lose them" (Johnson, 1985). This statement accurately conveys the difficulty grandparents have in defining their caregiving positions and depicts the uncertainty of how best to raise grandchildren with limited available resources. Navigating the complex welfare system adds considerable burden for grandparent caregivers, who often take care of their grandchildren with little or no assistance from other family members.

TANF is the single largest source of cash assistance for grandparents under age 65 who are caring for children (Mullen & Einhorn, 2000). However, TANF is often not enough to keep grandparent-headed households out of poverty. On average, 19% of grandparent-headed households were living in poverty in 1999 (Simmons & Dye, 2003). Children living in grandparent-headed households with no parents present are three times as likely to be receiving public assistance, but are also twice as likely to be living in poverty, as compared to children living with parents and grandparents (Fields, 2003). African American grandmothers and their grandchildren are especially likely to live below the poverty line and rely on public assistance to care for their grandchildren (Minkler & Fuller-Thompson, 2005; Casper & Bianchi, 2002; Casper & Bryson, 1998).

Age, race, gender, social class, labor force participation, and difficult family circumstances intersect to create multiple points of disadvantage among grandparent caregivers. Grandparent caregivers are susceptible to numerous economic hardships, including overcrowded and unsafe housing, insufficient food budgets, and struggles with Medicaid enrollment (Fuller-Thompson & Minkler, 2003; Bryson & Casper, 1999). Many of these grandparents may also be dealing with a host of difficult social issues, including death, divorce, domestic violence, and drug abuse. Indeed, the decision to "exchange a child for a child," particularly in the case of parental drug addiction, is emotionally devastating for grandparents who intervene for the well-being and safety of a grandchild (Harris, 2001). Family conflict, social isolation, and financial strain only add to the pressure that grandparents feel to save their families from dissolution, as well as rescue their grandchildren from the bureaucratic "stranger care" of the foster care system (Harris, 2001).

Foster care licensing requirements may exacerbate poor economic conditions among grandparent-headed households. Today, all states are required to provide the same payments to kin as they make for non-kin foster parents (*Miller v. Youakim*, 1979), and at least 40 states modify or waive licensing standards to accommodate relative caregivers (Leos-Urbel, Bess & Geen, 2000). However, the definition of foster kinship care differs dramatically across state lines, and states vary in their flexibility of how these families are treated (Geen, 2003). For example, the Adoption and Safe Families Act of 1997 restricts federal reimbursement of Title IV-E funds to states unless relatives meet the same licensing standards as non-relatives. This act places enormous pressure on states to treat relative and non-relative caregivers the same, although both groups may be dealing with widely different social and economic circumstances. In turn, becoming a licensed foster care provider is a daunting task for grandparent caregivers, many of whom are unaware of their eligibility or unable to meet state licensing requirements. Many grandparents are also simply unwilling to be involved in the child welfare system, afraid their decision may put their grandchildren at risk of being placed in a non-kin foster home if they are unable to comply with state standards (Jendrek, 1994).

TANF policies do not adequately reflect how the structure and function of families have changed, particularly the important role of extended family members, such as grandparents, who intervene for the well-being and safety of their grandchildren. The insufficient recognition of intergenerational families in welfare policies represents structural lag: the asynchrony between enacted social policies–which are often discussed and passed in the legislative "bubble" of Capitol Hill–and the increasing heterogeneity of family forms (Riley, Kahn, & Foner, 1994). Grandparents are often the "silent saviors" for families struggling with relationship, economic, and social instability (Creighton, 1991). As the stewards of these fragile families (Carlson, McLanahan, & England, 2004), grandparents should be included in the current discussion of welfare reform.

TANF: A POROUS SAFETY NET FOR AMERICA'S POOREST

One purpose of TANF, as specified by Section 401(a) of the Social Security Act, is "to provide assistance to needy families so that children may be cared for in their own homes or in the homes of relatives" (U.S Social Security Administration, 2005). Another purpose of TANF is, "to end the dependency on government benefits by promoting job preparation, work and marriage" (U.S. SSA, 2005). Funding for job training and adult education have been sizable portions of the federal block grant allocated to states. However, TANF programs that encourage financial solvency do not include special provisions for grandparent caregivers who may be unable to work. Work requirements are an example of how grandparent caregivers can be unfairly penalized for participating in the welfare system.

Work Requirements and Grandparent Caregivers

Work requirements are included as part of the Personal Responsibility and Work Opportunity Reconciliation Act (PWORA) without consideration for how compliance to these strict rules will affect grandparents who may not have been in the labor force for a long time or may be unable to work. Employment and training policies are one of the largest sites for the devolution of responsibility from federal to state agencies. However, the lack of coordination among state and local-level programs severely restricts job opportunities and job sustainability among older workers (Doeringer, Sum, & Terkla, 2002). Similarly, corporations' benefit packages often do not include the special needs of grandparent caregivers and their grandchildren. In a national survey of corporations, Generations United found that none of the businesses surveyed allowed grandparents to include grandchildren as beneficiaries on their employer-provided health insurance without legal custody, guardianship, or adoption (Biscarr, 2002). This survey also revealed that other employee benefits, such as child-care, family leave, and counseling programs, were inaccessible or inapplicable for grandparent caregivers' specific needs.

The "work first" philosophy of TANF has increased employment among low-income families, but often in jobs with low earnings, reduced mobility, and few, if any, health benefits. According to the Urban Institute's National Survey of America's Families, median wages for people leaving welfare in 2003 were $8.06 an hour, which has not increased since 1999 (Loprest, 2003). Similarly, a meta-analysis of 30 studies conducted by the Center for Law and Social Policy (CLASP) revealed that only one-quarter of people who leave welfare receive employer-sponsored health benefits (Strawn, 2004). Statewide programs that prepare welfare recipients for work, as well as safeguards to keep them in the labor force such as health care benefits, remain sorely under-funded. The lack of a supportive work environment may increase the recidivism rate for those who leave welfare, especially during times of economic recession (Andersson, Lane, & McEntarfer, 2004).

Although the effectiveness of work requirements continues to be heavily debated by welfare policy experts, a formal discussion of how these rules may affect grandparent caregivers has not been initiated at the federal level. Grandparents who are caring for children can apply for a "child-only" grant, in which children receive TANF assistance. In this case, grandparent caregivers would not receive any TANF benefits and would be exempt from federal work requirements. However, the child-only grant may not be suitable for poor grandparents who may need welfare benefits for themselves, as well as the children under their care. If grandparents choose to be a part of the family "assistance unit" and receive these benefits, they would be required to work at least 30 hours a week in most states (Urban Institute, 2002). Failure to comply with hourly work requirements without "good cause" would result in a possible discontinuation of TANF benefits and permanent ineligibility for the entire household (Mullen & Einhorn, 2000).

For example, only 28 states provide "hardship exemptions" for people 60 years of age and older, which excludes these grandparent caregivers from federal sanctions, such as work requirements (Urban Institute, 2002). States with a high proportion of grandparents as caregivers, such as California and New York, provide age-related work exemptions. However, the lack of age exemption in some states may disadvantage older grandparent caregivers, who must then choose between receiving TANF and adhering to federal work requirements, or not receiving any welfare assistance.

The Senior Community Service Employment Program (SCSEP), under Title V of the Older Americans Act, attempts to address the difficulties that older workers face in finding employment (AARP Foundation, 2005). However, work requirements add considerable burdens for grandparent caregivers for several reasons. First, many older grandparents, particularly women, have been out of the labor force for a long period of time and may have difficulty finding employment. Second, vocational training programs often prepare workers for occupations with low wages and little prestige (Minkler, Berrick, & Needell, 1999). Third, studies have revealed that grandparent caregivers often report worse health than others their age, including increased Activity of Daily Living impairments (ADLs) and depression (Minkler & Fuller-Thomson, 1999; Minkler, Fuller-Thompson, Miller, & Driver, 1997). Health problems, particularly psychological well-being, are dependent on contextual factors that often lead to intense and prolonged stress among grandparent caregivers, including crisis situations regarding the child's parents, grandchildren's emotional problems, financial difficulties, and isolation (Giarrusso, Feng, Silverstein, & Marenco, 2000). If forced to comply, work requirements would add considerable burden to grandparent caregivers, many of whom are already dealing with multiple social and economic stressors that may affect their physical and emotional health in the long run.

Marriage Promotion: What "I Do" Programs Don't Do for Grandparent Caregivers

Another reason TANF policies do not adequately address the unique needs of grandparent-headed households is their focus on strengthening marriage. One purpose of TANF, which promotes, "encouraging the formation and maintenance of two-parent families," has come into the spotlight in recent years, giving the federal government unprecedented authority over the private institution of marriage. Since the 1990s, every state has made at least one policy change or undertaken at least one activity designed to promote marriage in attempts to reduce divorce and non-marital childbearing (Ooms, Bouchet, & Park, 2004). In addition, both the House and the Senate have proposed over $1.5 billion dollars in the next five years to support an array of "marriage promotion" activities, including teenage pregnancy prevention, marriage education, and responsible fatherhood programs (U.S. House of Representatives, 2004). These programs are known collectively as the Healthy Marriage Initiative (HMI). The effectiveness of these programs for non-married couples has been brought into question in recent years (McLanahan, 2003). However, the impact of HMI programs for intergenerational families, such as grandparent-headed households, has not yet been addressed. A discussion of the historical impetus of encouraging marriage, as contained within U.S welfare policies, will shed light on how the passage of the HMI will affect grandparent caregivers.

Historically, from colonial Poor Laws to the passage of the Personal Responsibility and Work Reconciliation Act, the public sanctity of marriage has been emphasized as the "essential institution of a successful society which promotes the best interest of children" (PWORA, 1996). For example, "parental fitness" requirements, which were part of the Aid to Dependent Children program (ADC) in the Social Security Act of 1935, excluded unwed mothers who continued to have children out of wedlock from obtaining welfare benefits by declaring these homes unsuitable to raise children (Frame, 1999). Similarly, "man in the house" policies penalized unmarried, cohabiting women from receiving welfare benefits until 1968, when these rules were finally held unconstitutional (*King v. Smith*, 1968). These policies gave state and federal governments unchecked authority to dictate whether women were "deserving" of aid, depending on their reproductive choices and family arrangements. Current TANF legislation continues to include moral language that encourages or dissuades certain social behaviors. For example, family cap provisions in 23 states restrict unwed mothers from receiving additional welfare benefits if they continue to have children while on welfare (U.S Department of Health and Human Services, 2004a).

The recent interest in expanding marriage promotion funds stems from the belief that higher welfare benefits encourage "non-traditional" family values, such as single parenting, delayed marriage, and cohabitation. However, research has produced mixed results concerning the effects of welfare policies on family structure (Bitler, Gelbach, Hoynes & Zavodny, 2004). Most studies show little or no effect of welfare policies on women's marriage and childbearing decisions (Peters, Plotnick, & Jeong, 2001; Moffit, 1998). Despite the inconclusive evidence of the ability of welfare programs to prescribe social behavior, an inherent goal of welfare policy is to ensure the well-being of children, which policymakers often link to the preservation of married, two-parent families. Marriage education programs can be beneficial for both men and women, especially if they are educating people about domestic violence and promoting active fatherhood. Researchers have been touting the advantages of marriage for the healthy development of children for decades. In fact, hundreds of studies outline the benefits of marriage for families with children, including improved economic standing, positive psychological well-being, and increased educational and job opportunities (Waite, 1995; McLanahan & Sandefur, 1994).

There can be no doubt that there are benefits of the Healthy Marriage Initiative for some people, but these programs do little to serve grandparents and other relatives who take on the responsibility of caring for young children. Few programs exist at the federal level to ensure that grandparents remain employed, or provide support for those grandparents unable to work. Instead, individual states are responsible for providing these supportive programs. A portion of the HMI funds should be focused on the development and maintenance of educational programs, job training, and child-care, which would better serve grandparent caregivers. Similarly, some HMI funds should be reallocated to support directly grandparent caregivers who are unable to work. States are instrumental in the oversight and implementation of these social programs.

"LABORATORIES OF DEMOCRACY":
TANF AND STATE-LEVEL POLITICS

The "aging network" includes the Area Agencies on Aging, state units on aging (SUA), and community organizations. Both Area Agencies on Aging and state units on aging have been at the forefront of developing creative programs to address the needs of grandparent caregivers and their families. States have always played an integral role in shaping the amount and form of public aid for the poor. Even before the passage of PWORA, states were given waivers, or exemptions from federal regulations, in order to experiment with different ways of administering welfare programs. Proponents of welfare devolution claim that states, not the federal government, are better able to serve local constituents. According to this view, states serve as local, autonomous "laboratories" for the development of innovative and tailored social policies (Donahue, 1997). However, critics of welfare devolution argue that states have made TANF policies more restrictive in order to avoid becoming "welfare magnets" for the poor of neighboring states (Rom, Peterson, & Scheve, 1999). In this way, states may adopt welfare policies to compete with other states, rather than attempt to reduce poverty within state lines.

State-run welfare programs have significant administrative gaps that do not assist many grandparent caregivers with the multiple responsibilities associated with caring for children, such as health insurance, school enrollment and housing. Many of these complex issues cannot be addressed directly by the "aging network," spearheaded by state units on aging, because these organizations are not adequately equipped to provide assistance to intergenerational families. The AARP's Grandparent Information Center (GIC) is a good starting point for grandparent caregivers to find information on various caregiving issues, which potentially bridges these gaps (AARP, 2005). Similarly, Title I of the Kinship Caregiver Support Act, proposed by the Senate, is a program that would assist kinship caregivers in navigating through existing state programs and services. However, as policies currently stand, grandparent caregivers must maneuver through a variety of social service agencies, such as the Center for Medicare and Medicaid Services (CMS), Housing and Urban Development (HUD) and local schools, in order to receive necessary assistance.

Health Insurance Coverage

Children in grandparent-headed households are likely to have high rates of health problems, such as asthma, weakened immune systems, poor sleeping and eating patterns, physical disabilities, and attention deficit hyperactivity disorder (Minkler & Roe, 1996; Shore & Hayslip, 1994). These health problems make access to health services for grandchildren of paramount concern; however, approximately one in three children cared for by grandparents has no health insurance (Bryson & Casper, 1999). Access to health insurance may be impeded by several factors. The most pervasive barrier to obtaining health insurance is grandparents' lack of knowledge on how to obtain child health benefits. TANF requires a separate application for Medicaid and for the State Children's Health Insurance Program (SCHIP), and many grandparents may not be aware that eligibility for Medicaid and SCHIP does not require legal custody in most states (Bissel & Miller, 2004). Collaboration between statewide health departments and welfare agencies would provide grandparents with more information about health care options for themselves, as well as their grandchildren.

School Enrollment

Previous research on grandparents and school enrollment noted that the Elementary and Secondary Education Act (ESEA) did not include adequate provisions to ensure that state and local educational agencies would work with grandparent caregivers to alleviate difficulties in school enrollment (Smith & Beltran, 2000). Although ESEA was reauthorized as the No Child Left Behind Act in 2002 (NCLB), there have been no provisions to simplify the process of school enrollment for caregivers without legal custody, or any language that refers to non-parental caregivers in the bill. Two of the main purposes of the NCLB act are to maintain parental involvement and to expand educational resources for disadvantaged students, such as minorities, immigrants, and disabled children, as well as children from low-income families. However, children who do not live with their parents are not emphasized in the NCLB bill. The goal to provide equal opportunities and high-quality education for children must be emphasized in NCLB to include children living in intergenerational families.

Housing

Previous research shows that access to adequate and affordable housing is a problem for many grandparent caregivers (Fuller-Thompson & Minkler, 2003). Grandparent caregivers who cannot afford housing consistent with state regulatory laws may receive lower payments from child welfare agencies and may experience discrimination from Housing and Urban Development (HUD) officials, who may believe that grandparent caregivers without legal custody are ineligible for housing subsidies (Minkler & Odierna, 2001). Generations United, an intergenerational public policy organization, was instrumental in the passage of the LEGACY bill in 2003, which provided a demonstration housing program for intergenerational families, mandated training for HUD employees, and funded a national study of the housing needs of grandparent caregivers. However, current housing policies are out of step with the changing needs of families (Fuller-Thompson & Minkler, 2003; Cobb & Dvorak, 2000). Expansion of existing housing programs and increased collaboration between regulatory agencies regarding housing requirements and waiver eligibility will ensure that safe, affordable housing will be available for grandparents and their families.

WELFARE REFORM AND POLICY RECOMMENDATIONS

The National Family Caregiver Support Program (NFCSP), appended to the Older American's Act in 2000, provides caregiver support services administered at the state level. This program allocates funding for families caring for the elderly and children, with the purpose of alleviating the financial and emotional stresses that often accompany the caregiving role. Approximately 10% of the funds appropriated for the NFCSP can be used to provide services to grandparent caregivers. However, NFCSP as a stand-alone federal program is often inadequate for relative caregivers, particularly those without legal custody. The welfare "safety net" should be improved to include grandparent caregivers who are not reached by existing federal, state, and local programs. Several changes should be made to existing federal and state TANF programs so they are accessible to grandparents and their families:

1. *Expand TANF Goals to Include Grandparents Raising Grandchildren.* In recent years, the goals of TANF have focused more explicitly on family structure, rather than unemployment, as a major determinant of poverty among American families. TANF was written under the assumption that the formation of two-parent, married families will reduce welfare dependency. Intergenerational families such as grandparents raising grandchildren are omitted from the bill, despite that these families are disadvantaged by difficult, often insurmountable, social, and economic circumstances. Explicit language in TANF legislation recognizing the importance of intergenerational families would ensure that grandparent caregivers receive necessary assistance.

2. *Formalize State Exemption Criteria for Grandparent Caregivers.* As mentioned, federal work requirements have a negative effect on

older caregivers, who may have been out of the work force longer, are poorer, more likely to be disabled or in ill health, and who may possess fewer skills applicable in today's job market. All states should include formal exemption from work requirements for grandparents who are incapacitated, over age 55, ill, or disabled.

3. *Reevaluate Effects of the Healthy Marriage Initiative on Intergenerational Families.* To a large degree, welfare reform initiatives are taking shape under the rubric that healthy marriages are the key to reducing poverty. However, the Healthy Marriage Initiative (HMI) does not address the multiple causes of poverty, such as the reduced availability and sufficiency of skilled labor positions for welfare recipients. In fact, passage of the HMI would allocate *over three times more* money to marriage promotion and research than what was spent on job education and training in 2003 (U.S. Department of Health & Human Services, 2004b). This is money that is earmarked for purposes that will never reach grandparent caregivers. Similarly, the emphasis on two-parent married families skews the distribution of federal funds away from grandparent caregivers who may be in acute need of federal, state, and local assistance. HMI funds should be reallocated to preserve job training and educational programs that provide intergenerational families with a better chance of leaving welfare permanently.

4. *Close the Gaps in State "Aging Network" Services.* Statewide "aging networks" often do not have a way of coordinating local services such as health care, school enrollment, and housing services for grandparents responsible for their grandchildren. Grandparents may not be aware of particular services in their area or may be unclear whether they and their grandchildren are eligible to receive assistance. Efforts should be made to increase communication among local programs. The Brookdale Foundation, a non-profit organization, has funded "Relatives as Parents" programs (RAPP) in 42 states and is an example of how state and local agencies work in conjunction to provide services to grandparent caregivers (Brookdale Foundation, 2004).

CONCLUSION

The TANF bill contains the implicit assumption that *maintenance of the two-parent family is the only pathway to economic self-sufficiency.*

In this case, the two-parent family is viewed as a conduit through which married men and women can find and keep jobs and leave welfare successfully. This narrow interpretation of the family persists in federal welfare legislation, despite that a "family unit" is never explicitly defined in the TANF bill (U.S. House of Representatives, 2004). To date, welfare policies have not included adequate provisions for intergenerational families who are often faced with severe financial hardships and difficulties accessing necessary social services. Welfare legislation should include a broad definition of the family so that state-administered TANF programs reflect the needs of diverse family forms, such as grandparents raising grandchildren. Similarly, administrative gaps between state and local organizations should be bridged so that grandparents can readily access and utilize existing state and local programs. The promotion of an inclusive definition of the family within welfare policies will ensure that all families have the opportunity for a secure and prosperous future.

AUTHOR NOTE

Casey E. Copen, MPH is a PhD student at the University of Southern California in the Department of Sociology. The author would like to thank Lynne Casper and Phoebe Liebig for their helpful suggestions on earlier drafts of this manuscript. Address correspondence to: Casey Copen, 3715 McClintock Avenue, Los Angeles, CA 90089-0191 (E-mail: ccopen@usc.edu).

REFERENCES

AARP (2005). *Grandparent information center.* Available online: <www.aarp.org>.
AARP Foundation (2005). *Senior community service employment program.* Available online: <www.aarp.org>.
Andersson, F., Lane, J., & McEntarfer, E. (2004). *Successful transitions out of low wage work for TANF recipients: The role of employer, coworkers, and location.* Washington, DC: The Urban Institute.
Bengtson, V. L. (2001). Beyond the nuclear family: The increasing importance of multigenerational bonds. *Journal of Marriage and the Family, 63:* 1-16.
Biscarr, M. (2002). *Grandparents and other relatives raising children: Support in the workplace.* Washington, DC: Generations United.
Bissel, M., & Miller, J. L. (2004). *Using subsidized guardianship to improve outcomes for children: Key questions to consider.* Children's Defense Fund. Available online: <http://www.childrensdefense.org>.

Bitler, M. P., Gelbach, J. B., Hoynes, H. W., & Zavodny, M. (2004). The impact of welfare reform on marriage and divorce. *Demography, 41*(2): 213-236.

Brookdale Foundation (2004). *The relatives as parents program.* Available online: <http://www.brookdalefoundation.org>.

Bryson, K. R. & Casper, L. M. (1999). *Co-resident grandparents and grandchildren.* Current Population Reports P23-198. Washington, DC: U.S. Department of Commerce.

Carlson, M., McLanahan, S., & England, P. (2004). Union formation in fragile families. *Demography, 41*(2): 237-262.

Casper, L. M., & Bianchi, S. M. (2002). *Continuity and change in the American family.* Thousand Oaks, CA: Sage.

Casper, L. M. & Bryson, K. R. (1998). *Co-resident grandparents and their grandchildren: Grandparent maintained families.* Population Division Working Paper #26. Washington, DC: U.S. Census Bureau.

Cherlin, A. J., & Furstenberg, F. F. (1986). *The new American grandparent.* New York: Basic Books, Inc.

Cobb, R.L., & Dvorak, S. (2000). *Accessory dwelling units: Model state act and local ordinance.* Washington, DC: AARP Public Policy Institute.

Creighton, L. (1991, December 16). Silent saviors. *U.S News & World Report,* 81-9.

Doeringer, P., Sum, A., & Terkla, D. (2002). Devolution of employment and training policy: The case of older workers. *Journal of Aging & Social Policy, 14*(3/4): 37-60.

Donahue, J. D. (1997). *Disunited states: What's at stake as Washington fades and states take the lead.* New York: Basic Books.

Fields, J. (2003). Children's living arrangements and characteristics: March 2002. In *Current population reports* (P20-547). Washington, DC: U.S. Census Bureau.

Frame, L. (1999). Suitable homes revisited: A historical look at child protection and welfare reform. *Children & Youth Services Review, 21*(9/10): 719-54.

Fuller-Thompson, E., & Minkler, M. (2003). Housing issues and realities facing grandparent caregivers who are renters. *The Gerontologist, 43*(1): 92-98.

Fuller-Thomson E., & Minkler M. (2001). American grandparents providing extensive child-care to their grandchildren: Prevalence and profile. *The Gerontologist,* 41(2): 201-9.

Fuller-Thompson, E., & Minkler, M. (2000). The mental and physical health of grandmothers who are raising their grandchildren. *Journal of Mental Health & Aging, 6:* 311-323.

Geen, R. (Ed.). (2003). *Kinship care: Making the most of a valuable resource.* Washington, DC: Urban Institute Press.

Giarrusso, R., Feng, D., Silverstein, M., & Marenco, A. (2000). Primary and secondary stressors of grandparents raising grandchildren: Evidence from a national survey. *Journal of Mental Health and Aging, 6*(4): 291-310.

Goodman, C., & Silverstein, M. (2002). Grandmothers raising grandchildren: Family structure and well-being in culturally diverse families. *The Gerontologist, 42*(5): 676- 689.

Harris, S. C. (2001). *Relative strangers: An ethnography of grandmothers raising grandchildren in the Los Angeles county child welfare system.* Unpublished PhD dissertation, University of Southern California, Los Angeles.

Jendrek, M. P. (1994). Grandparents who parent their grandchildren: Circumstances and decisions. *The Gerontologist, 34*(2): 206-216.

Johnson, C. L. (1985). Grandparenting options in divorcing families: An anthropological perspective. In V.L. Bengtson & J.F. Robertson. (Eds.) *Grandparenthood.* (pp.81-96). Beverly Hills: Sage Publications.

King, V., & Elder, G. H. (1999). Are religious grandparents more involved grandparents? *Journal of Gerontology, 54*(6): S317-S328.

King v. Smith, 329 U.S 309 (1968).

Leos-Urbel, J., Bess, R., & Geen, R. (2000). *State policies for assessing and supporting kinship foster parents.* Washington, DC: The Urban Institute. Available online: <http://www.urban.org>.

Loprest, P. J. (2003). *Fewer welfare leavers employed in weak economy.* Washington, DC: The Urban Institute. Available online: <http://www.urban.org>.

Lugalia, T., & Overturf, J. (2004). *Children and the households they live in: 2000.* Census 2000 Special Report. Washington, DC: U.S. Census Bureau.

McLanahan, S. (2003). *Fragile families and the marriage agenda.* Working Paper 03-16-FF. Center for Research on Child Well-Being. Available online: <http://crcw.princeton.edu>.

McLanahan, S., & Sandefur, G. (1994). *Growing up with a single parent: What hurts, what helps.* Cambridge, MA: Harvard University Press.

Miller v. Youakim, 44 U.S. 125, 99 S. Ct. 957 (1979).

Minkler, M., & Fuller-Thompson, E. (2005). African-American grandparents raising grandchildren: A national study using the Census 2000 American Community Survey. *Journal of Gerontology, 60*(2): S82-S92.

Minkler, M., & Odierna, D. (2001). *California's grandparents raising grandchildren: What the aging network needs to know as it implements the National Family Caregiver Support Program.* Berkeley, CA: Center for the Advanced Study of Aging Services.

Minkler, M., Berrick, J. D., & Needell, B. (1999). *The impact of welfare reform on grandparents raising grandchildren.* San Francisco, CA: Public Policy Institute of California. Working Paper No.18.

Minkler, M., & Fuller-Thompson, E. (1999). The health of grandparents raising grandchildren: Results of a national study. *American Journal of Public Health, 89*(9): 1384-1389.

Minkler, M., Fuller-Thompson, E., Miller, D., & Driver, D. (1997). Depression in grandparents raising grandchildren: Results of a national longitudinal study. *Archives of Family Medicine, 6,* 445-452.

Minkler, M., & Roe, K. M. (1996). Grandparents as surrogate parents. *Generations, 20*: 34-38.

Moffitt, R. A. (1998). *Welfare, the family and reproductive behavior: Research perspectives.* Washington, DC: National Academies Press.

Mullen, F., & Einhorn, M. (2000). *The effect of state TANF choices on grandparent-headed households.* Washington, DC: AARP Public Policy Institute. Paper #2000-18.

Ooms, T., Bouchet, S., & Parke, M. (2004). *Beyond marriage licenses: Efforts in states to strengthen marriage and two-parent families.* Washington, DC: Center for Law and Social Policy. Available online: <http://www.clasp.org>.

Personal Responsibility and Work Opportunity Reconciliation Act of 1995. 42 USC 1305. § 101 (1996).

Peters, H. E., Plotnick, R. D., & Jeong, S. O. (2001). Discussion Paper #1239-01 *How will welfare reform affect childbearing and family structure decisions?* Institute for Research on Poverty. Madison, WI: University of Wisconsin. Available online: <http://www.irp.wisc.edu>.

Riley, M. W., Kahn, R. L., & Foner, A. (1994). *Age and structural lag: Society's failure to provide meaningful opportunities in work, family, leisure.* New York: John Wiley & Sons, Inc.

Rom, M. C., Peterson, P. E., & Scheve, K. F., Jr. (1999). Interstate competition and welfare policy. In S. F. Schram & S. H. Beer (Eds.) *Welfare reform: A race to the bottom?* Washington, DC: Woodrow Wilson Center Press.

Shore, R. J., & Hayslip, B. (1994). Custodial grandparenting: Implications for children's development. In A. Godfried and A. Godfried (Eds.), (pp. 171-218). *Redefining families: Implications for children's development.* New York: Plenum.

Silverstein, M., Giarrusso, R., & Bengtson, V. L. (1998). Intergenerational solidarity and the grandparent role. In M. Szinovacz (Ed.) *Handbook on grandparenthood.* (pp.144-158). Westport, CT: Greenwood Press.

Simmons, T., & Dye, J. (2003). *Grandparents living with grandchildren: 2000.* Washington, DC: U.S. Census Bureau.

Smith, C. J., & Beltran, A. (2000). Grandparents raising grandchildren: Challenges faced by these growing numbers of families and effective policy solutions. *Journal of Aging & Social Policy, 12*(1): 7-17.

Strawn, J. (2004). *Why Congress should expand, not cut, access to long term training in TANF.* Center for Law and Social Policy. Available online: <http://www.clasp.org>.

Urban Institute (2002). *Welfare rules database.* [Data file]. Available online: <http://urban.org>.

U.S. Census Bureau (2005). *Grandchildren under age 18 living in the home of their grandparents: 1970 to present.* Historical time series table CH-7. Available online: <http://www.census.gov/population/socdemo/hh-fam/tabCH-7.pdf>.

U.S. Department of Health and Human Services (2004a). *TANF: Sixth annual report to Congress.* Available online: <http://www.acf.hhs.gov/programs/ofa/annualreport6/ar6index.htm>.

U.S. Department of Health and Human Services (2004b). *TANF Financial Data.* Available online: <http://www.acf.hhs.gov/programs/ofs/data/index.html>.

U.S. House of Representatives, Committee on Ways and Means (2004). *2004 green book.* Washington, DC: Author.

U.S. Social Security Administration, Committee on Ways and Means (2005). *Compilation of the social security laws.* Available online: <www.socialsecurity.gov>.

Waite, L. J. (1995). Does marriage matter? *Demography, 32*(4): 483-507.

doi:10.1300/J031v18n03_13

State Policy Decisions in the 1990s with Implications for the Financial Well-Being of Later-Life Families

Gretchen J. Hill, PhD

Arkansas State University

SUMMARY. This study explores trends and patterns in states' policy decisions affecting the economic well-being of later-life individuals and families in the United States in recent decades, focusing on the 1990s. Rules were selected from the areas of inheritance, estate taxes, homestead exemptions, Medicaid eligibility, estate recovery, and filial responsibility. Results indicate an increasing use of a broad definition of family, one implying that spouses, the nuclear family, extended kin, step-relations, and sometimes in-laws constitute an ongoing collective whose members share economic resources and risks over their lives and beyond. Despite this global trend, states varied in their rules addressing intrafamilial financial obligations and families' accountability to states. While some seemed interested in facilitating the conservation of familial resources, others seemed willing to minimize public assistance while coercing kin into accepting financial responsibility for one another. Research was suggested to answer questions raised by this study. doi:10.1300/J031v18n03_14 *[Article copies available for a fee from The Haworth Document Delivery Service: 1-800-HAWORTH. E-mail address: <docdelivery@haworthpress.com> Website: <http://www.HaworthPress.com> © 2006 by The Haworth Press, Inc. All rights reserved.]*

[Haworth co-indexing entry note]: "State Policy Decisions in the 1990s with Implications for the Financial Well-Being of Later-Life Families." Hill, Gretchen J. Co-published simultaneously in *Journal of Aging & Social Policy* (The Haworth Press, Inc.) Vol. 18, No. 3/4, 2006, pp. 211-227; and: *Family and Aging Policy* (ed: Francis G. Caro) The Haworth Press, Inc., 2006, pp. 211-227. Single or multiple copies of this article are available for a fee from The Haworth Document Delivery Service [1-800-HAWORTH, 9:00 a.m. - 5:00 p.m. (EST). E-mail address: docdelivery@haworthpress. com].

KEYWORDS. Aging, elderly, family, policy, law, inheritance, Medicaid, estate recovery, filial responsibility

INTRODUCTION

Whether by long-standing arrangements or through recent trends in federal-state relations, many of the rules that contribute to elder and family policy in the United States are decided at the state level. A number of rules in these policy domains relate to both older individuals and the family, especially ones that address rights, expectations, and obligations of support, assistance, or property. While there is federal involvement in some areas where the states make policy choices, the trend toward program "devolution"–the federal government's transfer of transfer rights, powers, and responsibilities to states and local governmental units–has made many policies less uniform across the country. This study explores states' family-related elder policy decisions in the 1990s, focusing on those that can affect families' economic resources.

METHODS

An extensive review of law and policy studies published in recent decades helped to identify relevant state laws and regulations. A rule was defined as relevant to elder policy if it specified an age of 55 or older, or dealt with phenomena that tend to be more common in later life, such as, disability or death. Within elder policy areas, rules were deemed relevant to familial financial well-being if they directly or indirectly affected the resources owned by or available to the family as a whole, or to an individual by virtue of being a family member. Rules meeting these criteria were found in the following substantive areas: inheritance law, tax codes, debtor-creditor law, Medicaid regulations, estate recovery plans, and filial responsibility statutes.

Data were collected for 1990 and 1999, or only the latter for rules first appearing after 1990. For rules in domains with a long history of state control, 1960 data were collected in order to clarify trends. Several data sources[1] were used for each domain, triangulated by source in order to increase reliability. A state was coded as having a particular rule in an observation year based on the descriptions of state statutes, case law, and agency regulations in the data source materials.

Content analysis was used to classify rules. Three questions guided the classification: (1) Does the rule affect the number of familial economic resources, or access to resources, or shift them among different family members? (2) Does the rule obligate, encourage, limit, or prohibit certain behaviors of families or family members with respect to economic resources? (3) How are different categories of family members affected by the rule?

RESULTS AND DISCUSSION

Results of content and trend analyses are set out in Table 1. The number of states with each rule is set out by observation year. The rules listed in the table are explained in the context of discussing each policy domain. Rules range from those affecting economic resources of families having substantial assets, to rules aimed at families in financial straits. Also discussed are potential effects of the rules on later-life families, including extended family members.

Inheritance

Most Americans view the ability to pass on property–particularly to family–as a basic right (Shammas, Salmon & Dahlin, 1987). The practice of inheritance is held to play an important role in family well-being and to strengthen the family as an institution (Foster, 2001). Further, elderly individuals, especially those who are frail or disabled, may need the element of power that can come from the control over assets that inheritance law confers (Dobris, 1989). Inheritance has long been the province of the states, whose statutes contain both commonalities and rule differences (Hill, 1995; Shammas et al., 1987). Results of the trend analyses of 1960, 1990, and 1999 state inheritance laws suggested general patterns of change in recent decades.

Intestate Succession. When someone dies without a Will, intestate succession laws set out the division of assets. Historically, lineal heirs, such as children or grandchildren, received a larger share than a surviving spouse, but this pattern was gradually reversed over the past century (Hill, 1995; Leiter, 1999; Shammas et al., 1987). As Table 1 shows, priority of lineal inheritance decreased from about a half, to one-third, to a quarter of the states in 1960, 1990, and 1999, respectively. Some states went so far as to adopt "spouse-all inheritance" rules that either gave a spouse everything outright, or set a spousal minimum share at a dollar

TABLE 1. Number of States with Selected Rules in Selected Years

RULE	YEAR		
	1960	1990	1999
INHERITANCE LAWS			
Lineal inheritance given priority over spousal inheritance	24	17	13
Spouse-all inheritance in intestate succession formula	1	19	24
Intestate succession formula provides for reconstituted families	0	26	31
Spousal elective share is based on length of marriage	0	0	7
STATE TAX ON INTRA-FAMILIAL INHERITANCES [a]	44	20	13
HOMESTEAD EXEMPTION STATUTES	41	43	47
Generous[b] homestead exemption provision	6	6	17
MEDICAID LONG-TERM CARE SPOUSAL PROTECTIONS			
Uses federal maximum community spouse protected resource limit	na	16	23
Uses federal minimum community spouse protected resource limit	na	29	19
Community waiver program allows spend-down and/or Miller trusts [c]	na	-	38
ESTATE RECOVERY PLANS			
Estate recovery plan in place	1	18	46
Authorizes use of TEFRA liens to secure state's rights to property	na	3	13
Extends recovery beyond probate estate, as permitted by OBRA93	na	na	14
Covers more services than required under OBRA93	na	na	22
Hardship provisions include waiving recovery of homestead	na	na	24
FILIAL RESPONSIBILITY LAWS			
Adult child has obligation to support financially indigent parent	34	26	29
Child's obligation to parent may be used to limit government aid	15	22	26

[a] Estate or inheritance taxes other than the credit estate tax tie-in to federal estate taxes.
[b] Maximum exemption is at least $50,000. This figure was suggested for a homestead allowance under the 1969 Uniform Probate Code (Hill, 1995). A state's homestead exemption was considered generous if the value of exempt property was no less than this amount.
[c] Reliable data sources for rules prior to 1999 were not located.

value higher than the value of most estates (Hill, 1995). The prevalence of spouse-all inheritance increased from just one state in 1960, to 38% of the states in 1990, to about half the states by 1999.

In another trend, states have been adopting intestate laws that decrease the spousal share in step-family situations (Gary, 2000). First, most states with a spouse-all inheritance rule stipulate that it applies only when all of the deceased spouse's children are the surviving spouse's children. Second, other states have enacted intestate laws that decrease the spousal share if the deceased spouse has surviving children who are not children of the surviving spouse. Altogether, about 60% of the states adopted intestate succession rules recognizing reconstituted families by 1999.

Spousal Election. The "spousal election" statute gives a surviving spouse the right to claim a different share of estate property than whatever is bequeathed in the deceased spouse's Will. In 1991, the National Conference of Commissioners on Uniform State Law (NCCUSL), an advisory group of law professionals, suggested that if the amount that could be elected was contingent upon length of marriage, then family property divisions would be fairer in the increasingly common cases of later-life remarriages (Hill, 2003). By 1999, seven states had adopted NCCUSL's spousal election formula (see Table 1). Curiously, the rule takes a shotgun approach to dealing with increased longevity and the diversity in family forms. That is, it applies to all marriages and family types, rather than targeting remarriages or a specific age group. Moreover, those getting more when the spouse gets less are those named in the Will, who may not be family members.

Inheritance and Estate Taxes. Alongside federally-imposed estate taxes, nearly all states taxed inheritances during the past century and, having smaller tax exemptions, affected more families than the federal tax (Pechman, 1987; Sitarz, 1999). Periodic changes in the federal estate tax tended to be followed by changes in state taxes. In part, states' responsiveness has been due to a federal "credit estate tax" provision, also called a "pick-up tax," which creates a state-federal link. States opting to take advantage of the pick-up tax become entitled to a portion of any federal tax paid by estates administered in the state. By 1990 all states had instated the pick-up tax provision (Hill, 1995).

Just as federal estate tax codes have allowed ever-increasing amounts to be inherited tax-free, the trend at the state level has been a close parallel (see Table 1). In 1960 nearly 90% of the states imposed their own inheritance or estate taxes, not just a pick-up tax. By 1990 this had dropped to 40%, and then to a quarter of the states by 1999. Thus, entering the twenty-first century most states taxed only those estates subject to federal taxes. As a result of fewer independent state inheritance and estate taxes, and with no federal estate tax on spousal inheritances, plus a $675,000 federal exemption otherwise, only about 2% of families faced any estate tax liability (Kaplan, 2002).

Yet, the future of estate taxes is uncertain. Federal participation in the pick-up tax ends in 2005 under the Economic Growth and Tax Relief

Reconciliation Act of 2001 (EGTRRA), meaning that most states will collect no tax revenues from inheritances. EGTRRA repeals the federal estate tax altogether in 2010, but in 2011 EGTRRA "sunsets": it goes out of effect; federal tax law reverts to year 2000 rules, and the credit estate tax reappears (Klooster, 2003; O'Sullivan & Weaver, 2003).

Homestead Exemptions

Recognizing that the family home can be quite important to family financial well-being, most states have instituted a "homestead exemption" law to safeguard all or part of a homeowner's primary residence from creditors under stipulated conditions, usually in cases of bankruptcy or after the death of a family's income provider. Homestead exemption rights are considered so basic and important in some states that they are mandated by state constitution. Enabling families to keep their homes tends to decrease the likelihood that they will wind up on public assistance (Brown, 1997). In 1999 nearly all (94%) of the states had homestead exemption laws, up from 80% in 1960 (see Table 1). A few states' exemptions set no limit on the value of the homestead that could be protected, but most set limits ranging from a few hundred dollars to several hundred thousand dollars (Martindale-Hubbell, 1961-2000). During the 1990s, the number of states with relatively generous exemptions, defined as $50,000 or more (Hill, 1995), doubled from 9 to 18. Meanwhile, federal bankruptcy and Medicaid reformers have been trying to get a cap set on the value of homestead exemptions as they apply to their respective venues (Hynes, Malani, & Posner, 2004).

Medicaid and Long-Term Care

Inheritance laws and homestead exemptions might provide some insight into how states regard family members' needs, interdependencies, and expectations, but the rules might matter little to those who have few assets to hold onto, bequeath, or inherit. One area potentially important to the elderly and their families, whether of substantial assets or little means, concerns paying for long-term care. The elderly are particularly susceptible to conditions requiring long-term care. Private insurance is often inadequate or unaffordable, and most families are unable to cover the costs or provide the care on their own. Thus, many turn to Medicaid, the only government program that provides for extended long-term care, as the payer of last resort (Regan, 1995; Rein, 1996).

Medicaid was never intended to be a long-term care program for the elderly; it was to provide a safety net for persons of limited assets and income. Medicaid rules are exceedingly complex, and as the federal statute has given more responsibility and options to the states, interstate variation in programs has increased (Moses, Marohn-McDougall, & Moses, 2004). However, in every state many aspects of elders' and families' lives may be affected when care is needed and Medicaid assistance is sought. Those elderly who are unable to afford needed long-term care worry about whether they can qualify for Medicaid assistance, and if so, how family finances will be affected. The latter concern is largely based on two worries: the financial sufficiency of "well" family members, especially dependents, and being able to leave *something* for loved ones to inherit.

Older persons in poverty who need long-term care usually immediately qualify for Medicaid coverage as "categorically needy": those whose financial resources fall below limits set by their state. But, many nonindigent elderly qualify as "medically needy": those whose financial resources exceed state limits for categorically needy status, yet are insufficient to finance the costs of their medical care. Although states can extend medically needy coverage to any categorical group, the elderly have been the primary beneficiaries (Moses et al., 2004). The following areas include aspects of Medicaid that are most relevant to elderly needing long-term care.

Medicaid Spend-Down. Most states that allow people to become eligible under medically needy provisions require them to "spend down" their income and assets. States exempt certain items, such as a primary residence or a car, and non-exempt assets are used to pay care costs until assets have been reduced to allowable levels. Income over the maximum limit is spent down each month; the amount of income over the state limit must be used toward a beneficiary's medical care.

Spend-down can be a source of considerable concern to elderly persons facing the prospect of extended long-term care, particularly those with a "community spouse" who does not need care. Some Medicaid rules are aimed at preventing "spousal impoverishment" of the community spouse. One provision is the community spouse "resource allowance" setting out the value of a couple's assets that can be kept and still qualify the medically needy spouse for benefits. Maximum and minimum standards are set at the federal level, and states set their allowances within these limits (Day, 2002). In 1990, one-third of the states used the federal maximum resource standard; 58% used the minimum, and the remaining 10% established a standard in between the two (see

Table 1). In 1999, 46% used the maximum; 38% used the minimum, and 18% fell in between. Thus, during the 1990s, about a third of the states became more generous toward the community spouse.

Miller Trusts. Some states' Medicaid programs impose an "income cap" on eligibility. As a result, persons in need of long-term care with assets below resource allowance levels may remain ineligible for assistance due to their income levels. At one time, persons in this situation had few choices: Move to a state without the cap, rely on family and friends, or forego care (Estes, 1993). In 1993 the Omnibus Budget and Reconciliation Act (OBRA93) required income cap states to recognize qualified income trusts, or "Miller trusts," and to ignore income paid into them. The trust must be in place before applying for Medicaid so that the applicant is not receiving the income–the trust is. Trust funds help pay for the Medicaid recipient's long-term care costs; Medicaid picks up the slack, and after the recipient's death Medicaid can claim any remaining funds. A Miller trust essentially simulates income spend down, but many elderly residents of income cap states do not know about the option. Consequently, they make other arrangements for long-term care, thus saving the state hundreds of thousands of Medicaid dollars every year (Fleming & Curti, 1997).

Community Waivers. Originally, Medicaid's long-term care options were tied to institutional settings. In the 1980s, Congress gave the Health Care Financing Administration (HCFA), the federal agency administering Medicaid, the power to waive institutional care for approved state programs. Under "community waivers," states could develop plans for covering community-based services, such as in-home care or assisted living, to a certain number of qualifying people. Generally, both care recipients and the states benefit from community waivers. Most older long-term care patients prefer staying at home, and providing community care usually costs the state less than providing institutional care. By 1999, every state had at least one community waiver program, and although neither establishing a medically needy category nor allowing Miller trusts are required, three-fourths of the states did extend one or both provisions under community waivers (see Table 1).

Estate Recovery

As the review of states' Medicaid eligibility rules suggests, elderly persons needing long-term care can qualify for Medicaid coverage and still have substantial assets. Moreover, due to Medicaid spend-down exempt property rules and states' homestead exemptions, a Medicaid beneficiary is likely to die owning assets. Thus, those wishing to leave an inheritance to their loved ones may have the wish fulfilled. However, "estate recovery" policies might yet prevent inheritances from reaching intended beneficiaries. Under estate recovery, the states recoup some costs of financing long-term care under Medicaid by collecting from some recipient's remaining assets after she or he has died.

States always have had the option to recover their Medicaid costs, but until the 1990s they had little incentive to do so (Day, 2002; Miller, 1994; Zieger, 1997). Congress began encouraging estate recovery in the 1980s, hoping to curb Medicaid costs as they tried to balance the federal budget (Kinney, 1990). The 1982 Tax Equity and Fiscal Responsibility Act (TEFRA) aimed to give states greater access to assets of Medicaid recipients ages 65 or older (Escarce & Lavizzo-Mourey, 1990). For the first time, estate recovery rules were made explicit in federal law. Instituting estate recovery remained optional, but TEFRA did seem to prompt some states to act. By 1990 just over a third of the states had estate recovery plans (see Table 1).

TEFRA Liens. To facilitate the estate recovery process, TEFRA also gave states the option to use "TEFRA liens." The lien could be placed on any real property wholly or partly owned by an institutionalized Medicaid recipient, provided the patient was not expected to return home. The lien could not be enforced while the patient was living. After the patient's death, four situations would preclude a state from enforcing a lien upon the residence: (1) a surviving spouse, even if not living in the home; (2) a child under age 21, or blind or disabled child of any age, even if not living in the home; (3) an adult child who lives in the home and lived in the home at least two years prior to the Medicaid recipient's admission to the nursing home and provided care that postponed the nursing home admission; (4) a sibling who lives in the home if he or she lived in the home at least two years prior to the Medicaid recipient's admission to the nursing home. As a consequence, states may have to wait to effect recovery, but use of the lien would prevent the property from being given away, sold, or distributed to heirs not fitting the above categories, without the state first having an opportunity to make a claim (Kinney, 1990; Miller, 1994). But, by 1990, only three states used TEFRA liens (see Table 1).

OBRA93. OBRA93, mentioned in the discussion of Miller trusts, introduced three estate recovery rules with far-reaching implications for families in which an older individual received Medicaid benefits. First, receiving federal Medicaid funds would be contingent upon establishing an estate recovery plan. Second, recovery plans could define "estate" more broadly than "probate estate." A probate estate–consisting of inheritable property typically conveyed through a court procedure–usually excludes some assets, like those transferred by survivorship rights (e.g., joint tenancy, living trusts). Instead, states could seek estate recovery from a wide variety of assets in which the beneficiary had some ownership rights. Finally, OBRA93 lowered the age at which long-term care beneficiaries would be subject to estate recovery. States were instructed to recover costs for nursing home services, home and community-based services, and related hospital and prescription drug services expended on behalf of Medicaid beneficiaries ages 55 and over.[2]

Hardship Exemptions. OBRA93 directed states to establish procedures for foregoing estate recovery when it would cause "undue hardship." Federal analysts suggested excluding a family home from recovery when it was the primary remaining asset (Miller, 1994). Medicaid statutes already prohibited actions aimed at recovering a home if a surviving spouse, a dependent child, or other qualifying family member lived there, but once the situation changed–family members moved out, died, tried to sell the house, or altered ownership–the state could act (Zieger, 2001).

By 1999, all but four states had established estate recovery plans (see Table 1). Some states enthusiastically embraced estate recovery and chose aggressive methods to implement it, such as using TEFRA liens (Day, 2002). Some states established plans only after receiving warnings that federal funding would be withheld (Barnes, 2003; Shelton, 2004). West Virginia rebelled by trying to get the estate recovery portion of OBRA93 declared unconstitutional (*West Virginia v. Department of Health & Human Services*, 2002). However, most states showed ambivalence, such as setting up estate recovery plans, but doing very little to carry them out (Frank, 2003).

States' differing approaches to estate recovery are indicated by plan differences (see Table 1). Among the 46 states with estate recovery plans in place by 1999, fewer than 30% had instituted TEFRA liens. Just 30% used an expanded definition of estate property. Not quite half (48%) would seek reimbursement for more Medicaid-provided services than required under OBRA93. And, despite the ubiquity of state homestead exemption laws, just under half would waive recovery against a family home. As Medicaid estate recovery rules continue to be worked out by legislatures and the courts, there is very little interstate coordination (Dick, 2004; Frank, 2003; Miller, 1994).

Filial Responsibility Laws

Forty-five of the 50 states at some time in their histories have had "filial responsibility" laws articulating adult children's obligations financially to support their indigent parents (Jacobson, 1995; Warner, 2001; Wiesner, 1995). The number of states with such laws at any point in time has fluctuated widely over the past century, and the extent of their enforcement is unclear (Bulcroft, Van Leynseele, & Borgatta, 1989; Warner, 2001). Generally, an adult child's financial status is balanced against a parent's needs, such as food, clothing, shelter, and medical care. Typically, either a parent or the state may commence an action against a child. In some states, a child may counter demands for support by showing that the parent provided inadequate care when the child was a dependent minor, or otherwise failed in the parental role (Day, 1997; Spataro, 2000).

A 1960 study showed that 13 states were using their filial responsibility laws as a basis for reducing Old Age Assistance payments when adult children were available, whether or not children gave support (Schorr, 1960). But when it was established in 1965, Medicaid prohibited states from making any individual financially responsible for an applicant, except spouse for spouse, or parent for dependent child. As a result, states curbed their use of filial support laws (Moskowitz, 2001). Then, in 1977 Massachusetts proposed an experimental "family responsibility plan" that it hoped would help contain rising state Medicaid costs. Financially-able adult children living in the state would be obligated to help pay for a Medicaid-eligible parent's nursing home costs. Medicaid prohibitions were to be circumvented by obtaining a waiver. HCFA did grant the waiver in 1979, but the plan was dropped by the state without action (Acford, 1979).

Apparently, HCFA's 1979 decision for the Massachusetts plan was a harbinger of a policy reversal: In 1983, HCFA told states they could use their filial responsibility laws to require adult children to help pay long-term care costs of a Medicaid-eligible parent, or to recover Medicaid funds spent on a parent's care, provided their statute applied to all . public support programs in their state (Indest, 1988). A 1995 Medicaid bill that would have set this rule out in federal statute was passed by Congress, but vetoed by President Clinton (Fleming & Curti, 1995). Today, the rule remains explicit in HCFA's state Medicaid manual (Health Care Financing Administration, 2004).

Some states never rescinded filial responsibility laws passed over a century ago, but a number of states enacted new statutes in recent years.

As shown in Table 1, two-thirds of the states had filial responsibility laws in 1960. In 1990, this was down to just over half, but back up to nearly 60% by 1999. Of states with filial responsibility statutes in observed years, those with a statute of general applicability increased from 44%, to 85%, to 90%, in 1960, 1990, and 1999, respectively. This trend suggests some increasing interest in finding ways to shift the growing burden of long-term care costs from state programs to the families of those elderly needing care.

Many children already provide a great deal of support for elderly parents who need it. Imposing a legal financial responsibility in addition to family members' traditional caregiving roles seems unnecessary and unfair. Additionally, enforcing the laws seems impracticable, possibly illegal, and certainly would result in adult children's unequal treatment if the laws cannot be enforced with out-of-state children (Acford, 1979; Fleming & Curti, 1995).

OVERVIEW

Trends and patterns in the reviewed rules did reveal a fair amount of interstate variation through the 1990s in policies that can affect the economic well-being of later life individuals and families, even in areas subject to federal control. Yet, general patterns also were evident. One general pattern relates to how rules interconnect in their operation. Homestead exemption laws, along with Medicaid medically needy programs, protected resources, Miller trusts, and community waivers, have contributed to making Medicaid a safety net for elderly of various means if they require long-term care. And, OBRA93's estate recovery mandate to the states turned Medicaid's long-term care coverage into a quasi-loan program, at least for middle-class or more affluent older patients and families.

Moreover, by 1999 a sizeable minority of states complying with OBRA93, some aided by filial responsibility laws, had made familial assets more liable for covering older patients' long-term care costs, whether in lieu of Medicaid assistance, as a condition of Medicaid spend- down, or after a beneficiary's death when the state called in its "loan" through estate recovery. As a result, inheritance and estate tax laws might be less relevant in the future. Medicaid recipients' familial assets could be lessened by obligations to the state, and assets of those avoiding Medicaid may be depleted by care costs. Either way, these families could be left with very little inheritable property.

Another general pattern concerns implied definitions of the family. Many adopted rules seemed to place spouses, the nuclear family, extended kin, step-relations, and sometimes in-laws into a community of shared economic resources and financial risks extending over their lives and beyond. As noted, some Medicaid rules and filial responsibility laws could result in various family members' sharing financial responsibility for elderly kin. Trends in inheritance rules enhanced property entitlements afforded by the marital community, but also provided for heirs whose interests would conflict with spousal inheritance. And, by exempting most families from estate taxes, most 1999 state tax codes treated nuclear and extended kin as a family unit within which assets may be managed, exchanged, or shared without having to pay the state for the privilege.

Some states' policy choices implied a quite broad definition of family. For example, under some estate recovery plans the state can place liens on homes occupied by survivors of deceased Medicaid beneficiaries as security on repayment. Although recovery must be postponed until the death of the recipient's surviving spouse or disabled child, or until non-dependent children or siblings of the deceased no longer meet exemption requirements, states will continue monitoring the status of surviving family members and the recoverable property until recovery is permissible. As a result, heirs of the Medicaid recipients' surviving spouse, children, or siblings–even if those heirs are not legally related to the former Medicaid recipient, such as a surviving spouse's new spouse–may wind up in the family collective. Moreover, in states with inheritance or Medicaid rules that define joint tenancy or living trust property as part of an estate or as recoverable assets, any surviving joint owner or trust beneficiary, kin or not, may become part of the resource unit.

Looking at interstate variation in policy decisions, rule choices ran the gamut between facilitating and restricting access to Medicaid, between minimum and maximum protective resource limits, from aggressive to lackluster estate recovery plans, and more or less willingness to emphasize filial responsibility. Whereas lack of uniformity may not be a problem, some may find it disconcerting that state of residence can be a factor in later-life families' chances for financial security.

The parameters of this study did not include examining the extent to which interstate variations may or may not matter. This issue may be addressed by further research designed to identify intrastate patterns of rule configurations, and then to compare configuration patterns across states. Besides identifying which states appear to have the most family-friendly policies, results also may suggest whether a state's rules are coordinated so that its residents can anticipate their combined consequences, or if its rules seem disparate and fragmented, creating a policy quagmire.

Additional research might also be designed to answer questions like: If a state chose restrictive Medicaid qualifying rules, did it also set minimal resource protection limits, adopt aggressive estate recovery plans, and enforce filial responsibility laws? Results of further studies also might discern underlying principles or common goals that might guide a state's elder and family policy decisions, as well as suggest whether state financial well-being has a role. These and other questions raised by this study might be addressed by further trend and pattern analyses and other kinds of research on state policy processes and outcomes. As long as states continue to make important policy decisions in these areas, research on state policies should remain an important component of U.S. elder policy studies.

NOTES

1. Data sources for content and trend analyses: Inheritance law: Leiter, 1999; Martindale-Hubbell, 1960-2000; Shammas, et al., 1987; Sitarz, 1999. Estate taxes: Leiter, 1999; Martindale-Hubbell, 1960-2000; Pechman, 1987; Sitarz, 1999. Homestead Exemptions: Brown 1997; Hynes et al., 2004; Incorporate US, 2004; Leiter, 1999; Martindale-Hubbell, 1960-2000. Medicaid: Day, 2002; Frank, 2003; Health Care Financing Administration, 2004; Kaiser Foundation, 1992; Miller, 1994; North Carolina Long-Term Care Policy Office, 1999; Wiesner, 1995; Zieger, 1997. Filial Responsibility: Bulcroft et al., 1989; Garrett, 1979; Indest, 1988; Jacobson, 1995; Moskowitz, 2001; Narayanan, 1996; Schorr, 1960; Walters, 2000; Warner, 2001.

2. As an interesting side note, there is good evidence that the age change actually came about through a clerical error (*c.f.* Rein, 1996).

AUTHOR NOTE

Gretchen J. Hill, PhD, is Associate Professor of Sociology in the Department of Criminology, Sociology, & Geography at Arkansas State University. She also is an advisor and instructor for the university's interdisciplinary graduate certificate program in Aging Studies. Her research areas include state family and elder law and policy, filial responsibility expectations of adult children and elderly parents, and the well-being of adults in nontraditional relationships. Dr. Hill can be contacted at the University at P.O. Box 2410, State University, AR 72467 (E-mail: ghill@astate.edu).

REFERENCES

Acford, J. P. (1979). Reducing Medicaid expenditures through family responsibility: Critique of a recent proposal. *American Journal of Law & Medicine, 5*(1): 59-19.

Barnes, A. (2003). An assessment of Medicaid planning. *Houston Journal of Health Law & Policy, 3*: 265-299.

Brown, W. H. (1997). Political and ethical considerations of exemption limitations: The "opt-out" as child of the first and parent of the second. *American Bankruptcy Law Journal, 71*: 149-215.

Bulcroft, K., Van Leynseele, J., & Borgatta, E. F. (1989). Filial responsibility laws: Issues and state statutes. *Research on Aging, 11*: 374-393.

Cimini, C. N. (2002). Welfare entitlements in the era of devolution. *Georgetown Journal on Poverty Law & Policy, 9*: 89-134.

Day, P. (1997). The abandonment defense to a claim for parental support. *Journal of Contemporary Legal Issues, 11*: 380-387.

Day, T. (2002). About Medicaid coverage of long-term care. *Long Term Care Link.* Available: http://www.longtermcarelink.net/about_medicaid.html [2004, June 12].

Dick, D. L. (2004). The impact of Medicaid estate recovery on nontraditional families. *Florida Journal of Law & Public Policy, 15*: 525-557.

Dobris, J. C. (1989). Medicaid asset planning by the elderly: A policy view of expectations, entitlements and inheritance. *Real Property Probate & Trust Journal, 24*: 1, 5.

Escarce, J. J., & Lavizzo-Mourey, R. (1990). Recipients' estates: A source of revenue for Medicaid? *Annals of Internal Medicine, 112*: 725-756.

Estes, C. L. (1993). *The Long-Term Care Crisis: Elders Trapped in the No-care Zone*, Newbury Park, CA: Sage.

Fleming, & Curti, Professional Law Corporation (1995). Medicaid reform: "Family responsibility" laws. *Elder Law Issues, 3*(25). Available: http://www.elder-law.com [2001, July 12].

Fleming, & Curti, Professional Law Corporation (1997). Too much income? Medicaid may still be an option. *Elder Law Issues, 3*(49). Available: http://www.elder-law.com [2001, July 12].

Foster, F. H. (2001). The family paradigm of inheritance law. *North Carolina Law Review, 80*: 199-273.

Frank, J. C. (2003). How far is too far? Tracing assets in Medicaid estate recovery. *North Dakota Law Review, 79*: 111-145.

Garrett, W. Walton. (1979). Filial responsibility laws. *Journal of Family Law, 18*: 793, 798-99.

Gary, S. N. (2000). Adapting intestacy laws to changing families. *Law & Inequality, 18*: 1-81.

Gilbert, N., & Van Voorhis, R. A. (Eds.). (2003). *Changing Patterns of Social Protection*. New Brunswick, NJ: Transaction.

Health Care Financing Administration. (2004). General financial eligibility requirements and options: Treatment of contributions from relatives to Medicaid applicants or recipients. *State Medicaid Manual*, § 3812 (02-83). Available: http://www.cms.hhs.gov [2004, October 1].

Hill, G. J. (1995). Inheritance law in an aging society. *Journal of Aging & Social Policy, 7*: 57-83.

Hill, G. J. (2003). Finding fairness in U. S. family law. *Social Thought & Research, 25*: 193-216.

Hynes, R. M., Malani, A., & Posner, E. A. (2004). The political economy of property exemption laws. *The Journal of Law & Economics, 47*(1): 19-44.

Incorporate US. (2004). Basic homestead exemptions by state. Available: www.incorporate-us.com [2004, December 29].

Indest, G. F., III. (1988). Legal aspects of HCFA's decision to allow recovery from children for Medicaid benefits delivered to their parents through state responsibility statutes. *Southern University Law Review, 15*(2).

Jacobson, R. M. (1995). Americana Healthcare Center v. Randall: The renaissance of filial responsibility. *South Dakota Law Review, 40*: 518-545.

Kaiser Commission on the Future of Medicaid. 1992. *Medicaid at the Crossroads.* Menlo Park, CA: The Henry J. Kaiser Family Foundation.

Kaplan, R. L. (2002). Crowding out: Estate tax reform and the elder law policy agenda. *The Elder Law Journal, 10*: 15-46.

Kinney, E. D. (1990). Rule and policy making for the Medicaid program: A challenge to federalism. *Ohio State Law Journal, 51*: 855-916.

Klooster, T. J. (2003). Repeal of the death tax? Shoving aside the rhetoric to determine the consequences of the Economic Growth and Tax Relief Reconciliation Act of 2001. *Drake Law Review, 51*: 633-665.

Leiter, R. A (Ed.). (1999). *National Survey of State Laws* (3d ed.). Farmington Hills, MI: The Gale Group.

Martindale-Hubbell. (1961-2000). *Law Digests* (Vol. 8, Eds. 92-131). Summit, NJ: Martindale-Hubbell, Inc.

Miller, M. A. (1994). Your money for your life: A survey and analysis of Medicaid estate recovery programs. *Thomas M. Cooley Law Review, 11*: 581-611.

Moses, S. A., Marohn-McDougall, A., & Moses, D. V. (2004). *The Realist's Guide to Medicaid and Long-Term Care.* Seattle, WA: Center for Long-Term Care Financing.

Moskowitz, S. (2001). Filial responsibility statutes: Legal and policy considerations. *Journal of Law & Policy, 9*: 709-733.

Moskowitz, S. (2002). Adult children and indigent parents: Intergenerational responsibilities in international perspective. *Marquette Law Review, 86*: 401-455.

Narayanan, U. (1996). The government's role in fostering the relationship between adult children and their elder parents: From filial responsibility laws to...what? A cross-cultural perspective. *Elder Law Journal, 4*: 369.

North Carolina Long-Term Care Policy Office. (1999, Aug. 31). Comparing state Medicaid recovery efforts. Long-Term Care Policy Office with the Division of Medical Assistance, Department of Health and Human Services, North Carolina. Available: http://www.dhha.state.nc.us/aging/estate.htm [2000, May 29].

O'Sullivan, T. P., & Weaver, S. T. (2003). Planning for Kansas death taxes in 2003: A "notice-able" difference. *The Journal of the Kansas Bar Association. 72* (9): 28-41.

Pechman, J. A. (Ed.). (1987). *Federal Tax Policy* (5th ed.). Washington, DC: Brookings.

Regan, S. P. (1995). Medicaid estate planning: Congress' ersatz solution for long-term health care. *Catholic University Law Review, 44*: 1217-1267.

Rein, J. E. (1996). Misinformation and self-deception in recent long-term care policy trends. *Journal of Law & Politics, 12:* 195-340.

Schorr, A. L. (1960). *Filial Responsibility in The Modern American Family. An Evaluation of Current Practice of Filial Responsibility in the United States and the Relationship to it of Social Security Programs.* Washington DC: U.S. Department Of Health, Education & Welfare, Social Security Administration, Division of Program Research.

Shammas, C., Salmon, M., & Dahlin, M. (1987). *Inheritance in America from Colonial Times to the Present.* New Brunswick, NJ: Rutgers University Press.

Shelton, P. (2004). Estate recovery: The sleeping giant is waking up. Long-term Care Consultants (September 1). Available: http://www.ltcconsultants.com [2004, Dec. 27].

Sitarz, D. (1999). *Laws of the United States: Wills & Trusts.* Carbondale, IL: Nova.

Spataro, A. (2000). "Prodigal parent" as a defense to proceedings brought to require support from a child. *Journal of Contemporary Legal Issues, 11:* 385-388.

Walters, J. (2000). Support: Pay unto others as they have paid unto you: An economic analysis of the adult child's duty to support an indigent parent. *Journal of Contemporary Legal Issues, 11*: 376-379.

Warner, J. L. (2001, January 8). 29 states that may hold a child responsible for parental care. *NextSteps.* Available: http://www.nextsteps.net/articles/87.asp [2001, July 12].

West Virginia v. Department of Health & Human Services, 289 F.3d 281, 283-84 (4th Cir. 2002).

Wiesner, I. S. (1995). OBRA '93 and Medicaid: Asset transfers, trust availability, and estate recovery statutory analysis in context. *Nova Law Review, 19*: 679-733l.

Zieger, J. M. (1997). The state giveth and the state taketh away: In pursuit of a practical approach to Medicaid estate recovery. *The Elder Law Journal, 5*: 359-393.

doi:10.1300/J031v18n03_14

Index

BOOK ORDER FORM!

Order a copy of this book with this form or online at:
http://www.HaworthPress.com/store/product.asp?sku= 5894

Family and Aging Policy

___ in softbound at $19.95 ISBN-13: 978-0-7890-3374-1 / ISBN-10: 0-7890-3374-7.
___ in hardbound at $39.95 ISBN-13: 978-0-7890-3373-4 / ISBN-10: 0-7890-3373-9.

COST OF BOOKS _____

POSTAGE & HANDLING _____
US: $4.00 for first book & $1.50
for each additional book
Outside US: $5.00 for first book
& $2.00 for each additional book.

SUBTOTAL _____

In Canada: add 6% GST. _____

STATE TAX _____
CA, IL, IN, MN, NJ, NY, OH, PA & SD residents
please add appropriate local sales tax.

FINAL TOTAL _____
If paying in Canadian funds, convert
using the current exchange rate,
UNESCO coupons welcome.

❑ BILL ME LATER:
Bill-me option is good on US/Canada/
Mexico orders only; not good to jobbers,
wholesalers, or subscription agencies.

❑ Signature _____

❑ Payment Enclosed: $_____

❑ PLEASE CHARGE TO MY CREDIT CARD:

❑ Visa ❑ MasterCard ❑ AmEx ❑ Discover
❑ Diner's Club ❑ Eurocard ❑ JCB

Account #_____

Exp Date_____

Signature_____
(Prices in US dollars and subject to change without notice.)

PLEASE PRINT ALL INFORMATION OR ATTACH YOUR BUSINESS CARD

Name

Address

City   State/Province   Zip/Postal Code

Country

Tel   Fax

E-Mail

May we use your e-mail address for confirmations and other types of information? ❑Yes ❑No We appreciate receiving
your e-mail address. Haworth would like to e-mail special discount offers to you, as a preferred customer.
We will never share, rent, or exchange your e-mail address. We regard such actions as an invasion of your privacy.

Order from your **local bookstore** or directly from
The Haworth Press, Inc. 10 Alice Street, Binghamton, New York 13904-1580 • USA
Call our toll-free number (1-800-429-6784) / Outside US/Canada: (607) 722-5857
Fax: 1-800-895-0582 / Outside US/Canada: (607) 771-0012
E-mail your order to us: orders@HaworthPress.com

For orders outside US and Canada, you may wish to order through your local
sales representative, distributor, or bookseller.
For information, see http://HaworthPress.com/distributors

(Discounts are available for individual orders in US and Canada only, not booksellers/distributors.)

Please photocopy this form for your personal use.
www.HaworthPress.com   BOF06